GREGG CHARLES FISHER
IS JOINED BY SOME OF AMERICA'S LEADING
CFS EXPERTS TO CREATE TODAY'S MOST
COMPREHENSIVE, UP-TO-DATE VOLUME ON
CHRONIC FATIGUE SYNDROME

**Paul R. Cheney, M.D., Ph.D.**
The Cheney Clinic, P.A.
Charlotte, North Carolina
❖

**Nelson M. Gantz, M.D., F.A.C.P.**
Chairman, Department of Medicine
Chief, Division of Infectious Diseases
Polyclinic Medical Center
Harrisburg, Pennsylvania
❖

**David C. Klonoff, M.D., F.A.C.P.**
Clinical Professor of Medicine
University of California at San Francisco
❖

**James M. Oleske, M.D.**
Director, Division of Allergy,
Immunology and Infectious Diseases
University of Medicine & Dentistry
New Jersey Medical School

"Enlightening...anyone who reads this book will better understand
this perplexing syndrome."
— **Janet C. Bohanon, former co-director,**
**National CFS Association**

*Please turn this page for more acclaim for*
CHRONIC FATIGUE SYNDROME...

---

### Also by the Author

*Chronic Fatigue Syndrome:
A Victim's Guide to Understanding, Treating, and
Coping with this Debilitating Illness*

# CHRONIC

## A comprehensive guide to symptoms, treatments, and solving the practical problems of CFS

# FATIGUE

GREGG CHARLES FISHER
with contributions by Paul R. Cheney, M.D., PH.D.,
Nelson M. Gantz, M.D., F.A.C.P.,
David C. Klonoff, M.D., F.A.C.P., and James M. Oleske, M.D., M.P.H.

# SYNDROME

**WARNER BOOKS**

A Time Warner Company

Copyright © 1997 by Montco
All rights reserved.

Warner Books, Inc.,
1271 Avenue of the Americas, New York, NY 10020
Visit our Web site at
http://pathfinder.com/twep

W A Time Warner Company

Printed in the United States of America
First Printing: August 1997
10 9 8 7 6 5 4 3 2 1

Library of Congress Cataloging-in-Publication Data

Fisher, Gregg Charles.
    Chronic fatigue syndrome : a comprehensive guide to symptoms, treatments, and solving the practical problems of CFS / Gregg Charles Fisher, with Paul R. Cheney. . . [et al.].
        p.   cm.
    Includes index.
    ISBN 0-446-67268-8
    1. Chronic fatigue syndrome.   I. Cheney, Paul R.   II. Title.
RB150.F37F569   1997
616'.047—dc20                                         96-28333
                                                            CIP

Book design by Dianne Pinkowitz
Cover design by Tom Tafuri

This book is lovingly dedicated
to my precious Shawn,
the woman who is
my wife and my life,
and to
Mary, Bernard, Caren, Eric,
John, and Lou,
my dearly loved family:
No one embodies the true measure
of love more than you.

# Contents

# Foreword

Modern medicine has given us an air of near invulnerability. Day after day, the media brings us news of the latest "wonder drug" or miraculous surgical technique. After all, we can replace bones and joints, transplant kidneys and livers, even implant artificial teeth in our jaws and lenses in our eyes. The post–World War II generation has never known the summer scourges of polio or the mass quarantines of tuberculosis. Our concerns are the ills of advancing age: cancer, stroke, heart attacks.

Small wonder that the chronically ill are studiously ignored by the chronically well, particularly those in the prime of life. This social isolation can add an intolerable burden to an already limited lifestyle. Fortunately, the recent political mobilization of the physically challenged, culminating in the Americans with Disabilities Act, has resulted in greater accessibility to transportation and public facilities. Still, the United States is one of the few industrialized nations without a national health plan, so health-care costs that continue for decades keep most of the chronically ill well below the federal poverty level. The social services that might lighten the burden are all too often inaccessible to those most in need. The very effort to maintain life and limb often precludes the nourishment of heart and soul. New relationships are forestalled and existing ones are strained, often to the breaking point.

The author of this book, Gregg Fisher, has struggled with this type of crisis. Taken ill while still in graduate school, trying to maintain and nurture a relationship with his wife-to-be,

Shawn, he was faced with uncertain prospects of health, career, finances, and family. Many of us who have encountered similar situations have had no guidance as to how to proceed with our lives, or how to view our cloudy futures.

This book is the very personal story of one man's journey into night. It's a saga of bewilderment, faith, despair, and hope. As with all stories of chronic illness, it's a work still in progress, but it has some wonderful lessons to teach and may serve as a wellspring of inspiration for all.

Specifically for those afflicted with this ailment, known variously as chronic fatigue syndrome, CFIDS, myalgic encephalomyelitis, neuromyasthenia, or post-viral fatigue syndrome, this book contains a wealth of information, in terms that are made clear to the layperson. The medical contributors are Drs. Anthony L. Komaroff, Nelson M. Gantz, David C. Klonoff, James M. Oleske, and Paul R. Cheney, nationally recognized researchers and highly respected members of their profession.

As a fellow sufferer from this illness, and one who has spoken to many hundreds of others, I endorse this book wholeheartedly, and with great affection.

Robert Landau
Founder and Adviser
New Jersey CFS Association

When peace, like a river,
Attendeth my way,
When sorrows like sea-billows roll;
Whatever my lot, Thou hast
Taught me to say,
It is well, it is well
With my soul.

# Preface

As I continue to hear from people who suffer with chronic fatigue syndrome, I never cease to be amazed at the complete and utter devastation visited upon their lives. The letters I have received and the stories I have heard are all living testimonies to the relentless cruelty of this vicious illness. Though I try to respond to everyone, I often find myself at a loss about what to say. What words can I employ to encourage or comfort? What can I offer to ease others' suffering? I can say, "At least our illness isn't fatal," but that is like telling a man who is lost at sea that he should be grateful he isn't being eaten by sharks. I can say, "Researchers are working tirelessly for a cure," but that does nothing to relieve others' pain now.

Each person, sharing a common malady yet unique in his or her suffering, is filled with such pain and anguish that my soul cries out to God for them. My prayer is that he will touch these precious and courageous people in some very real way, as he has done for me. That is why a verse from my favorite hymn, "It Is Well with My Soul" opens this preface. It expresses, in ways I never could, my greatest source of strength and peace: my faith in God. From corresponding with many of you, I know this is true for you as well.

As my health has improved from some of the treatments mentioned in this book, however, I now look forward to the opportunity to share something more than mere consolation. Ever since I first became ill, I have recorded my experiences and reflections with the hope of someday putting them together in a book that would minister to others.

My goal, then, is to share the information that will help you understand, treat, and cope with this syndrome. This book, however, is not merely a compendium of impersonal information about CFS. For knowing about an illness without understanding how that illness affects the whole person is like knowing the statistics on hunger without understanding that people are dying of starvation. In this book I present information about CFS from my perspective as a sufferer and as the husband of a CFS sufferer as well. By showing how this illness has affected me and my family and how we have coped with and treated it, I hope to demystify CFS for you and to suggest ways of easing the pain and frustration of living with this syndrome.

What I will share with you is my personal experience and what I have learned along the way. CFS is an illness unlike any most people have ever heard of, let alone had. It's not like the flu—forty-eight hours of bed rest won't cure it— nor can it be eradicated with medications. Not yet. My only escape from this specter that haunts my every waking moment is sleep, and yet never is rest the victor. I awake to a day as difficult as the one before it.

If you have read the first version of this book, I hope that the years between editions have given me a fresh perspective that will translate into new insights for you. This is why each chapter begins with a quotation taken from the previous version. I have learned much about CFS and about how to cope with it, insights I consider it a privilege to share with you in the pages that follow.

In closing, please remember that I am not a doctor and cannot make a diagnosis or even recommend treatments. While this book was written with the help of some of the most prominent doctors involved in CFS research, it is intended solely to help you better understand and cope with CFS. Therefore, you should always consult your doctor before assuming a diagnosis of CFS or trying any treatment.

# CHAPTER ONE

# Our Story Continues

*Our nightmare began in January of 1982. I was twenty-four then and attending Trinity Evangelical Divinity School, in a northern suburb of Chicago, with the dream of becoming a minister. Just three months earlier I had met Shawn, the woman who was to become my wife. We were instantly attracted to each other, and our relationship blossomed into a lifetime commitment—one that truly tested our vow to stand by one another for better or for worse. Our road has not taken us on the typical couple's pilgrimage toward marital bliss. For most of our dating life and all of our married life, we have both been afflicted with chronic fatigue syndrome (CFS).*

I wrote that opening paragraph to the first edition of this book nearly ten years ago, and I can hardly believe that I am once again sitting down to continue the tale. Could it possibly be fifteen years since I first became ill, a decade and a half of my life lost forever to this insidious disease? Where has the time gone? What has happened to all my earlier hopes and dreams? The years pass so quickly now, a seemingly unending blur of sickness and pain. Dates and events, even one as momentous as the day I became ill, rarely impress themselves upon my consciousness anymore. Is this a normal function of getting older or has CFS so integrated itself into my being that that day in January of 1982 no longer stands out as one of the defining moments of my life? I have no way of knowing.

All I know is that I am sick and it feels like I have been so forever. To be quite honest, since I no longer remember what it truly feels like to be free of CFS I have no gauge by which to measure how "normal" feels. How do I determine what these past years would have been like without CFS? My first instinct is to say they would have been infinitely better than the life I have had, but upon further reflection I am not positive that is the case. There is a young woman in our church who actively ministers to those around her, has three beautiful children, a loving husband, and many friends; she also has cancer, and no more than six weeks to live.

We can never be sure what would have been in store for us if we had traveled a different path; things could have been better but they also could have been worse. The only thing I do know for sure is that who I am as a person has been permanently altered by my ordeal. The decisions I have made and the paths I have wandered have all been influenced by CFS and, for better or worse, it has transformed me forever. Like it or not, it has become as much a part of who I am as my name. In other words, it is part of what defines me. Therefore, to know who I am you have to know about my illness, you have to know my story.

The beginning of my struggle with chronic fatigue syndrome was on a weekend trip to Minnesota. Shawn and I were visiting some of her family and friends when I became sick with what I assumed was the flu. It's not all that uncommon for students to wear themselves down until they become ill, so other than ruining my weekend, there was nothing remarkable about the experience. I recovered enough to attend classes on Monday, and by the end of that week I was feeling much better.

At about that time Shawn too became ill—and her illness did not seem like a minor case of the flu. As the days passed, it became apparent that she was suffering from something far more severe. Every time I saw her she seemed to be dragging, as if living were a burden. She was exhausted all the time and slept constantly. She wasn't just too tired to wake up for her morning classes; she was too tired to wake up for her evening classes. She suffered unbearable headaches as well as a horribly painful sore throat, the kind that makes you think twice before enduring the pain of swallowing. She also found it difficult to think clearly, making studying impossible. In a word, her life was miserable.

Shawn somehow muddled through the next couple of weeks, but at great personal cost. It was obvious that her health was deteriorating, and I too began to feel ill. My symptoms were not as severe as Shawn's, but we both realized that they were too similar to be coincidental. And while we had no idea what we were suffering from, we knew it was considerably worse than the flu. The school nurse recommended that we be tested for mononucleosis. This seemed like such a logical diagnosis, I was certain that the blood tests were merely a confirming formality. I was wrong. The results of those blood tests ushered in the most emotionally turbulent four months of my life. Shawn tested positive for mononucleosis. I did not.

All my instincts told me I had the same illness Shawn had, but the blood tests disagreed. After more testing and ruling out other possible diagnoses, my only logical alternative was to believe that I was not seriously ill. In this era of medical marvels, it never even crossed my mind that blood tests may not be able to detect a serious illness. In my eyes, the medical establishment was infallible. If I truly did have mononucleosis, or some other serious illness, surely my doctors would have known.

I tried to convince myself that I was simply exhausted from my schoolwork, denying my illness in the hope that it would go away. I was so afraid of being seen as a hypochondriac that I didn't even discuss my illness with anyone else. I totally disregarded the pleas of my body for rest. As a result, my symptoms worsened.

Trapped in a bewildering world of conflicting emotions, I pushed myself to the point of exhaustion because I didn't think I had the right to be ill. Yet at the same time, I could feel my health deteriorating with each passing day. My studies suffered and my grades fell. My self-esteem was eroding as surely as my health as I blamed myself for my inability to ignore a "minor" illness. Meanwhile, Shawn's health plummeted to an indescribable depth of suffering, her pain so intense that her attempts to conceal it were to no avail. Every breath required a monumental effort of will. The pain and pressure in her head were incessant. She staggered around as if in a stupor, with barely enough stamina to eat, let alone attend classes. Most of the time she slept. But sleep only postponed the inevitable suffering until the next day. It never rejuvenated her, only numbed the pain for a few hours. This was a time of desperate need for Shawn, and there was nothing that I could do to help her.

Amazingly, despite all we were enduring, one thing we never even considered was dropping out of school. At the time we had an unquestioning faith in the medical system; since no doctor told us we needed complete rest, we felt we had no choice but to struggle on. Goals like graduating on schedule seem terribly unimportant now, but at that time we had no way of knowing what we truly needed. Also at work within us was a belief in our own invincibility. We were young, and felt that anything in life could be conquered if only we were tough enough. Vulnerability was alien to us. The strong were supposed to be immune to pain and weakness; only the frail succumbed.

In the end, the innate wisdom of our bodies prevailed. We could ignore the warning signals no longer. Two weeks before the end of the winter quarter we both left school. Often the full impact of an illness is not realized until it forces you into submission. When I went home, I collapsed from exhaustion. I hardly remember a thing from that time because I slept over sixteen hours a day, every single day, for six weeks. And during the eight hours I wasn't sleeping, I did nothing but rest.

Shawn also slept during most of this time. When she awoke, it took all her strength to walk the ten feet from her bedroom to the living room couch. She was too ill to watch TV or listen to the radio. At times she even had to close the living room curtains because the sight of any activity—even of birds building their nests or squirrels foraging for food—exhausted her as if she were doing the work herself.

After six straight weeks of rest we somehow managed to drag ourselves back to school. We really believed we would be well within a few weeks and that if we could just push through for a while, we wouldn't have to miss a whole quarter. The timetable I had imposed on the next three years of my life depended on finishing all of my classes in sequence. Rather than risk my schedule, I risked my health.

Even our doctors didn't advise against returning to school. Shawn and I were both told that these types of infections rarely last longer than a few months and that it would only be a matter of time until we were well. At that time, neither we nor our doctors knew that a chronic mononucleosis-like illness was even possible. And while my doctor could not say I had the same illness as Shawn, he could not rule it out either. Unfortunately, returning to school completely negated the benefits of the previous six weeks of rest.

The one positive result of my return to school was that I gained one of the most valuable insights I have ever learned: It can hurt just as much to love someone who is suffering as it does to suffer yourself. It may hurt in different ways, but the pain is no less intense. During all the years of my illness, my greatest anguish has come not from my own illness, but as a result of Shawn's. I had built up defenses to distance myself from my own pain, but hers was like an unerring arrow that could quickly and accurately find its way into the target of my heart.

We somehow finished the quarter and went our separate ways for the summer. I had the chance to work as a youth pastor at the Calvary Evangelical Free Church in New Jersey, a wonderful opportunity I just couldn't refuse. I wanted this experience so desperately that I didn't make the wise decision.

Rather than trying to work so hard, I should have listened to my body and rested the entire summer.

The more I tried to be tough and push myself, the worse I felt. My situation came to a head about halfway through the summer. My throat was so swollen and painful I could hardly talk. My entire body ached. I was exhausted, dead on my feet, and finally I collapsed. I had to resign my position because I was totally incapacitated.

Fortunately, my family doctor recognized how serious my condition had become, and had heard of other doctors who were dealing with symptoms much like mine. Drs. Alan Matook and James Oleske concluded that I was suffering from an illness known at the time as chronic mononucleosis. There was no effective treatment to be offered, but what a tremendous relief it was to have a doctor identify my illness and give a name to my affliction!

Unfortunately, Shawn's experience with doctors that summer was not as good as mine. After she explained that she had been extremely ill for the last six months, her first doctor advised her to gargle with salt water and predicted she would be well in two weeks. Her next doctor had the gall to tell her that she wasn't really ill, that she was just afraid of exerting herself. Later, though he hadn't seen her in $1\frac{1}{2}$ years, he informed Social Security that she was not disabled and did not deserve benefits. Even when she sent him journal articles on CFS by respected researchers, which included descriptions of her symptoms, he refused to believe. Instead he wrote his final diagnosis in bold letters across her chart: *Depression*. Naturally, Shawn did not return to these doctors. In fact, thinking there was no relief available, she stopped seeing doctors entirely.

To this day, as a result of both our experiences, I vacillate between condemnation and praise of the medical profession. Until I saw how Shawn's doctors treated her, I did not realize how fortunate I was to have found sympathetic, informed doctors. While they might not have known what I was suffering from, they at least believed I was suffering. I realize that we cannot expect doctors to be medical encyclopedias, aware of everything there is to know in the field of medicine, nor can we expect them to discount the possibility of hypochondriacal patients. But it is not too much to expect doctors to reach a middle ground and to treat seriously those patients who are truly ill.

In the fall we attempted to continue our education, but in January, one year after we first became ill, we no longer had the strength to carry on. I remember coming back to my dorm room and bursting into tears. I had not defeated this illness; it had defeated me. We both withdrew from classes and returned to our parents' homes.

I do not remember very much of the next few months. That time of my life was lived unconsciously. Shawn's family, however, was quite busy. They realized that they would have to take matters into their own hands if they were to learn anything about this illness. Her father spent hours at the library doing computer searches for any reference to a chronic type of mononucleosis.

They also called doctors and research facilities looking for information. Their search eventually led them to Dr. Stephen Straus and his research coordinator, Janet Dale, of the National Institutes of Health. The NIH is our nation's research hospital, located just outside of Washington, D.C., a huge facility with over fifty separate buildings and an annual budget in the billions. It also has one of the largest medical libraries in the world. People from all over the country are treated there, and since the NIH mainly researches unusual diseases, patients, who must apply to be admitted, are treated free of charge.

Our first visit lasted four days. We went through a battery of tests and were asked many questions. Dr. Straus was very kind, but told us there was no cure for our illness. He would, however, keep us in mind when they began researching possible treatments. Naturally we left there discouraged. We had hoped that we would hear the words "We will soon have a cure" rather than "This is just something you will have to learn to live with." Nonetheless, it was a tremendous relief to learn that due to Dr. Straus's interest in this syndrome, one of the greatest research facilities in the world not only believed in our illness, but was actually taking part in CFS research. We became frequent visitors to the NIH, but between hospital stays we tried everything we could think of—home remedies like aloe vera juice and a bitter-tasting beef-and-wine tonic, diets, vitamin therapies, moderate exercise programs, chiropractic, and many different medications—all in the hope of finding that elusive cure. Nothing helped.

It was because I was on a special diet during one of my trips to the NIH, and had lost a considerable amount of weight, that Dr. Straus was able to feel enlarged lymph nodes in my abdomen. They were so enlarged he became alarmed and sought the opinion of another doctor. Upon examination, they both felt that, though the chance was slight, it was possible I might have cancer. They had seen five patients with the same presentation and blood results as mine. Although there were some differences between us, one had developed cancer. I was stunned. Fear and dread hung over me like a dark cloud. Despite all I had been through with CFS, I was not prepared to face the possibility of my own death. For the first time in my life I felt completely alone.

I was finally broken. I had struggled through so many emotional stages with this illness. In the beginning there was total denial. I kept pushing myself because I would not admit that I was ill. When I could no longer deny the existence of my illness, my denial had become resistance: There was not an illness in the world I couldn't master—it would only be a matter of time until I was well. But as time dragged on, resistance had slowly become desperation. Having exhausted everything that mainstream medicine had to offer, I tried almost any treatment that had even the slightest chance of being effective, even some rather outlandish ones.

With this terrifying news, desperation quickly slid into despair. In one fell swoop, I had to face not only the possibility that I might not get well, but also the possibility that I might not live. My identity as an "ill person" was now complete. The faint flicker of hope I had for so long been fighting to keep kindled was now extinguished.

Yet, while the news was the worst I could possibly hear, I was, ironically, almost glad to hear it. At least with a diagnosis of cancer, no one could doubt that I was truly ill. After all, cancer is a relatively common disease that anyone can understand and empathize with. Until then, I hadn't understood how desperately I needed to be believed, to hear the sympathetic words, "You are truly ill," instead of the skeptical "Are you truly ill?" A part of me was willing to risk the ravages of cancer just so I would no longer have to explain my affliction or defend myself against the implication that I was lazy or crazy. I wasn't looking for pity. I just wanted the recognition and respect that other seriously ill people receive. I was subjected to a battery of tests for cancer—blood work, X rays, ultrasound, a CAT scan, a bone scan using radioactive isotopes, and others. The most painful was a bone-marrow biopsy, and I'm sure my fear that my incurable and interminable illness had spawned a more deadly disciple must have intensified the pain. I remember lying on the operating table and thinking how just two years earlier I had been perfectly healthy and looking forward to a fulfilling life. And as I endured pain greater than any I had known, I was shaken by my recognition of how radically my life had been altered by CFS. If there has been a low point in my struggle with this illness, that was it.

In the end there was no sign of cancer, but I realize now that the threat of cancer had a profound influence on my way of thinking about my life as a victim of CFS. Having been faced with the threat of a terminal illness, I began to understand how precious life is, even life with a chronic illness. I realized that I could no longer wait until a cure was found; I would have to learn to live as best I could with this illness even though I might not be able to live fully.

This new perspective, this determination, made possible something Shawn and I had been postponing for so long: our marriage. By then we had learned the value of rest in harboring our most important resource, our strength. We also had a support network of friends and family who were willing to help us over the financial hurdles. On the first of September, 1984, we were finally married, and time has proven what we then only suspected: that our emotional need for one another outweighed any possible difficulties marriage could ever present.

Our first year of marriage was, of course, more difficult than the average couple's. Between the two of us, we barely comprised one person. Taking care of our basic needs, such as cooking and cleaning, required all our strength and energy. We lived like nomads, staying in the homes of friends and relatives. Shawn once figured that, between moving and our trips to the NIH, we packed our bags an average of every two weeks that year.

The reason we made so many trips to the NIH was to take part in experimental treatments. I vividly remember the last treatment I received at the NIH. My arms were jabbed with IV needles, sometimes as many as ten times in one day. As I started reacting to the treatment, I became nauseous and vomited. I broke out into a cold sweat with alternating episodes of chills and fever. My whole body ached to the point where I broke down and cried, wondering how I could possibly hope to cope with this illness when I could barely cope with a possible cure. I was afraid to continue with this treatment because of its side effects, while at the same time afraid that the drug might not take effect.

Because of their often painful side effects and uncertain results, I've never felt comfortable submitting myself to experimental treatments. But oftentimes with complex illnesses such as ours, they offer the only chance at some relief. Thus, I undergo them, learning to walk a careful line between sensible optimism and naive hope. I need my optimism to maintain my determination, but frankly, I am terrified of hope, which is so easily dashed to pieces on the rocks of reality. In fact, the one time I seriously contemplated suicide was because I let my hopes get the upper hand.

I was under the care of a physician who boasted that he knew exactly what was wrong with me and guaranteed that I would be well enough to return to school in a few short weeks. Wanting desperately to believe him, I foolishly let my guard down and allowed my hopes to soar. After a month of costly and painful tests and treatments, he casually informed me that there was nothing more he could do and would I please leave because he was expecting another patient. No apologies, no explanations.

Abandoned not only by the doctor, but also by my own sustaining sense of hope, I fell into a depression—exacerbated, I suspect, by the medication he had given me—that brought me to the brink of suicide. Fortunately, I stopped taking the medication and began to recover from my depression. I was able to work through my suicidal feelings without acting upon them, but the experience has left its legacy. Whether for good or for ill, I resist opening myself up to the extremes of feeling, both other people's and my own, and I am especially cautious never to be vulnerable to the perils of unreasonable hope.

In fact, having any type of hope became increasingly difficult. When the first edition of this book came out it was entitled *Waiting to Live* because there was no aspect of my life or my dreams that CFS hadn't frustrated. At that time, I was practically bedridden and therefore considered the title terribly appropriate. Not only was I not feeling well, but I was also beginning to wonder if anything could ever change that condition. Most readers who were severely debilitated appreciated the title as a truthful portrayal of the impact of CFS. Others, especially those who had enough strength to resist many of the life-changing burdens of CFS, felt that the title represented psychological surrender. That a seemingly homogeneous patient group can have such diametrically opposed reactions to a book title reminded me that even though we may share a common syndrome, we are all uniquely affected by it. We may suffer with the same illness, but how we cope with and treat that illness varies from person to person.

If the severity of one's illness does truly affect the quantity and quality of one's hope, then I was pretty much running on empty. For a period of a couple of years I stopped trying treatments, attending support groups, or having anything to do with CFS. I wouldn't even read the CFS newsletters or watch the news when they covered the illness. I needed a break from this sickness, and since I couldn't do it physically, I had to do it psychologically.

I had gone through the stages of denial, resistance, desperation, and despair. I had stood up to the illness, learned about it, and tried everything I could to rid myself of it. Then I began the final stage of my emotional pilgrimage with CFS—acceptance. It is true that for many years, I had already worked very hard to accept this illness. I learned to cope with my new limitations and grieved the loss of my hopes and dreams. But I later discovered that acceptance entailed much more. True acceptance meant redefining my life and finding emotional balance. I needed to carve out a life for myself that included a debilitating chronic illness. It seemed to me that my CFS was not going to go away, and I could no longer allow myself to be obsessed with finding a cure. I needed to spend my energy redefining my purpose and goals, finding God's strength in my weakness.

In other words, I no longer spent my limited strength trying to eradicate CFS, but on finding ways to minimize its impact on my life. Feeling so completely overcome by this illness, it was not an easy process separating myself from myself, as if I were a pair of Siamese twins, to find the good when the bad is so prevalent. But, to maintain my sanity, there were periods during each day when I had to try to do just that. I needed to train myself to focus on the positive, no matter how mundane, and accept myself just as I was.

The impetus for this change hit me during what should have been one of the proudest moments of my life, the publication of *Chronic Fatigue Syndrome* by Warner Books. Becoming an author was hardly the experience I expected. I was surprised at how very little it did to raise my self-esteem. For example, I thought it would make me feel more comfortable in social situations to be able to respond "I'm an author" when asked the inevitably difficult question, "What do you do?" However, there was no comfort in telling strangers that my only book was about a strange and belittled malady that had ruined my life, all the while I was looking healthy. It was also extremely difficult to feel any sense of purpose or accomplishment because the subject I wrote about was the thing I despised the most in my life. Just when I should have felt great, I felt terrible. I was mired in a pit of emotional denial and suppression. I had attempted to have an identity as an author, trying to deny that I was someone afflicted with a chronic illness, yet all the while suppressing the painful emotions I suffered because of my chronic illness. The combination of these conflicting emotions created a strange amalgam in me. I was slowly losing the ability to know what I was truly feeling, and I was becoming consummate at feeling nothing at all. I was drowning in a sea of emotional and spiritual emptiness, and I no longer felt as if I had the strength to swim.

Therefore, though I never gave up wanting to get well, I realized that it was more important to deal with the emotional difficulties caused by not being well. By necessity, my focus shifted away from physical healing toward psychological, spiritual, and emotional healing. Shawn and I began attending a weekly prayer meeting that met near our apartment. Most weeks we barely dragged ourselves to the meeting, and our contributions to the rest of the group were pretty minimal. Week in and week out for a period of over two years, the people in this little group faithfully prayed for Shawn and me, bathing us in God's love and compassion. There were nights we cried and nights we laughed. Sometimes we felt God's healing touch and other times we didn't feel a thing. However, we found it tremendously healing to be consistently prayed for, especially since we often felt too weak to pray for ourselves. It was a very special and restorative time.

I also discovered counseling during this period. I must confess that Shawn had to drag me to my first appointment, but it wasn't very long until I was a very appreciative participant. I was fortunate to be blessed with gifted, caring counselors who recognized the connection between body and mind but never felt compelled to blame the ailments of the body solely on the mind. This was significant because it allowed me the freedom to be open and honest about seeking ways I could improve my condition, without feeling the need to defend the legitimacy of my illness.

Often I gained great insight into why I am the person that I am. I learned why I react the way I do, and why certain things are difficult for me to deal with. This helped me to cope better with my illness because I soon began to recognize two very important things: One, total control over one's circumstances, even for healthy people, is an illusion; and two, while I couldn't control my circumstances, I *could* control my reaction to them. That's not to say that positive thinking encouraged me to overcome CFS completely, but rather that insightful thinking enabled me to minimize the impact of this syndrome, at least to some extent.

I realize that this is a sensitive area, especially to patients who have been accused of psychologically causing their condition. We are not neurotic; we are suffering from a very real illness. However, any chronic illness has a psychological impact, and obtaining tools to minimize those effects can be very therapeutic. For example, there is a new branch of medicine called psychoneuroimmunology that studies the interactions among the brain, the endocrine system, and the immune system, because science has long realized their interdependence. Every aspect of the body is interrelated. Whether you have a cold or cancer, what you think and feel has some impact on how your illness progresses. Students tend to get more illnesses during finals, when stress is higher. And laughter has been shown to increase production of important illness-fighting cells.

Having been unable to control my body physically, I found it very therapeutic to gain some measure of control psychologically. For now, the pain of my illness is a given, but the effect that pain has on who I am can be mitigated to some degree. This illness is so unpredictable, affecting me in different ways depending upon the day, that gaining some semblance of control over my life became crucial. Sometimes just expressing how I felt was all I needed. Many times, my counselor was just someone who listened—sharing no new insights, just caring.

The key to all this is not looking at psychological wellness as a means to an end, but an end in and of itself. If I regard emotional wellness as the way I am going to be healed, then I will suffer despair and hopelessness if my health is not restored. If I look upon it as beneficial in its own right, then any resulting health benefits are just icing on the cake.

This time I spent restoring my spirit was incredibly healing for me. It renewed my sense of hope and optimism so that I was once again willing to try some new treatments. I tried a medicine called kutapressin, a liver extract that is supposed to have a modulating effect on the immune system. I had heard that some people with CFS had experienced improvement with it, but I must confess I tried it more or less on a lark. After so many failures I did not dare to suppose that it would make more of a difference than any other treatment I had tried. But, thank the Lord, I was wrong. This was the first medicine that ever truly made a significant, sustainable difference in my symptoms. I went from being 15 percent functional to being 30 percent functional, obviously not a cure but the only major improvement I had ever seen. A year later, Shawn also tried kutapressin and her sick, poisoned feeling improved, as did her cognitive abilities. She also no longer felt as much muscle weakness or fatigue.

Not being a doctor, I can't say why kutapressin helped Shawn and me when so many other treatments had failed. Nor can I say that it will help other CFS patients with equal effectiveness. It seems to me that the medicine, in and of itself, is quite beneficial, but I also believe that a number of other factors were involved, not the least of which was good timing. I truly feel that it was the right time for me to be on this medicine. My illness had stopped spiraling downward a few years before, and I had reached a plateau—though I was not getting any better at least I was not getting any worse. Therefore, I think my body was ready to begin the healing process.

After all, we are highly individualistic when it comes to our rate of recovery from illness. Just as some people get colds for twenty-four hours and others for forty-eight, our bodies respond differently to stresses and infections. Some people heal right away and others take a long time. Therefore, I am not sure that if I had tried this same treatment three years earlier it would have had the same impact. It might have; I just have no way of knowing. This is important, because we typically accept or discount treatments based on how effective they are in other people. But before we do, we should take into consideration whether or not those people are in a similar stage of their illness as we are.

As kutapressin increased our level of functioning, Shawn and I felt that maybe we would be able to notice improvement from some of the therapies we had tried in the past—therapies whose impact may have been too small to be noticed when we were so sick, but now might prove beneficial. Therefore, we went to a physical therapist who started us on a mild exercise program. In the beginning, I actually felt worse from the exertion, but over time I built up my stamina and endurance so that I found exercise very beneficial. The key is to listen to your body. We started out for thirty seconds on an exercise bike with no tension, and found that difficult. So proceed slowly!

We also began eating better and taking vitamins, minerals, and special supplements. This contributed to a greater sense of well-being. We also tried treatments for our sleep disorders and found tremendous benefit from a better night's sleep.

In addition, we found relief in attending to some of the non-CFS conditions that had developed since we became ill. For example, I began suffering from allergies, and Shawn developed an unusual problem that caused her to become light-headed and weak whenever she stood up or tried to do anything. She went to the Mayo Clinic in Rochester, Minnesota, where she was given a battery of tests that determined she had a defect in her autonomic nervous system, which controls the heart rate and blood pressure. Since this visit, researchers have found that many CFS patients develop similar problems with their blood-pressure regulation. This is usually diagnosed as neurally mediated hypotension.

To help her improve this condition, Shawn's doctor recommended that she wear support stockings that compressed her legs to help alleviate the pooling of blood in her feet. She also was given an exercise regimen to strengthen her circulatory system, which may have been weakened from deconditioning. In addition, she was told to increase her intake of salt, which helps ease the stress on the circulatory system.

I am still not well, but I am so much better from the treatments I've described in this book that I feel like a new person. I am still not as functional as I would like to be, nor can I sustain activity for any great length of time, but instead of the illness overcoming me I feel as if I am overcoming the illness.

Shawn and I strive to live each day as best we can. As difficult and painful as this illness is, we try to enjoy what life has to offer. We appreciate the simple pleasures and are grateful for the love we share with each other and with those around us.

Through the long years of this illness, we have had to struggle every day with our affliction. As the years go by, we are more determined than ever to remain strong. The saying "Time heals all wounds" is true, not because wounds, like sand castles, wash away with the first tide, but because in time you learn to survive your wounds.

Give yourself the time to learn to live with your wound. Shawn and I have managed it, and you can too. Hope comes not from seeing what is, but from dreaming of what might be.

# Symptoms

*The pain and sickness I experience is debilitating, but very little of my suffering is ever witnessed by the outside world. People don't see me when I'm having horrible days. They see me only for brief periods of time when I have rested enough to act as normally as possible. The next few days, when I am home alone, I suffer the unwitnessed consequences of that activity. Ironically, while I perceive my effort to silently endure the pain of my illness as noble, others misconstrue it to mean I am not really suffering. I am afraid that many people, because of their unfamiliarity with CFS and its often unobservable symptoms, tend to see me as either a hypochondriac or a malingerer.*

So much has changed with this illness since I first became ill, in fact not even the name is the same. But one thing that hasn't changed is the collection of vague and nondescript symptoms that comprise and define this syndrome. So many of the physical problems caused by CFS, such as fatigue or malaise, appear at best unobservable and at worst insignificant. I invariably look better than I feel, and to many physicians my symptoms seem to have no correlation to any objective physical findings because routine blood work or physical exams do not reveal any abnormalities. In other words, there is nothing I can do to verify my condition, which only adds to the emotional and psychological burdens imposed by any chronic illness.

While there are many other diseases, such as AIDS or MS, that are not completely understood, I know of no other ailment whose associated unknowns have been used so blatantly to attack the credibility of those who suffer with it. I realize that I have an unusual illness, and that my "normal" appearance makes it hard for others to respect the severity of my suffering. I also realize that there will always be people who judge with their eyes rather than with their minds, but I have come to the point in my life where I no longer waste precious energy trying to defend myself to these people. To them, my symptoms will always seem more like a crutch, masking psychological problems, than a cry of pain caused by a very real sickness. However, until there is a diagnostic test for CFS, symptoms remain the only method by which we can truly characterize and describe this insidious illness.

In this chapter, I will try to relate not just what the symptoms are, but how they impact our lives. I hope this serves two purposes: first, to give others the smallest inkling of the tremendous burden CFS imposes; and second, I wish to convey to those readers who feel isolated and alone that there are others who know what you are going through, who feel what you feel.

Much of what I describe is based on Shawn's and my experiences. It's important to remember that no one has every symptom, nor is every symptom necessary for diagnosing CFS. Some people experience a particular symptom all the time, while others experience it intermittently. Certain symptoms occur cyclically, for instance one week out of every month, while others occur randomly. Also, the severity of the symptoms varies from person to person. Many people with CFS are totally disabled, while others are merely annoyed. Typically, the severity of a symptom will be exacerbated by an increase in activity—the more you do, the worse you feel. Remember also that some of the symptoms I describe may not sound very debilitating. In fact, at one time or another, almost everyone experiences such symptoms as fatigue or headaches. However, degree is the key word here: CFS fatigue is to end-of-the-day tiredness what lightning is to a spark.

Looking back over the fifteen or so years I have been ill, I have noticed that very few of my symptoms have remained completely the same. Over time, and with the help of some treatments I will be describing, the ferocity of my symptoms has subsided. Instead of feeling as if they are destroying me, I feel as if now they are "merely" damaging me, not a small difference to anyone who suffers from this painful illness. To provide even more hope, I know of people who have improved to the point where their illness has subsided to being nothing more than a nuisance. Therefore, as you read my descriptions of the symptoms Shawn and I have suffered over the years, please remember that they represent some of the worst CFS has to offer. I am thankful that I no longer feel horribly ill all the time. I am hopeful that the worst is over, only a painful memory and not a daily reminder.

I mention this not only to encourage those who are severely crippled by CFS, but also to reach out to those whose symptoms were never that severe. You don't need to have experienced everything I did in order to justify your suffering in anybody's eyes. Suffering is suffering no matter what its form or severity. I realize that it is a part of human nature to compare ourselves with others—the first thing students do when they get a test back is to compare their grades with the people sitting next to them. However, it can be terribly self-destructive to do this with an illness. Other people's symptoms are not a yardstick by which to measure the severity of your own illness. When you understand this, you free yourself to acknowledge your own pain without feeling guilty that others may be more ill.

## FATIGUE

This is by far the most common symptom experienced by people with CFS. While fatigue is a common condition for the average American, the fatigue of a CFS sufferer can't be compared to that of a healthy person. It transcends anything I had ever experienced before I became ill. Not one moment goes by that I don't feel exhausted. I often feel like the Titan Atlas holding up the world—except that rather than easily bearing its enormous weight, I am weakly crushed beneath it. My fatigue is not only physical; it is mental, emotional, spiritual, and wearying beyond imagination.

I yearn for the simple pleasure of restful and refreshing sleep. Instead, though I am forced to rest and sleep a full two-thirds of my life, I feel just as exhausted when I wake up in the morning as I did when I went to bed. It is misery to go through each day as exhausted as the day before, to go to sleep every night knowing I am not going to feel rejuvenated when I awake, to regard my bed as a prison because that is where I am sentenced to spend most of my life.

For an outsider trying to understand why my fatigue is so debilitating, I can only liken it to the Chinese water torture. One day of fatigue, like one drop of water, does not seem terribly tormenting. But the unending presence of fatigue, like the incessant flow of water drops, is torturous. Anyone can withstand the strain of exhaustion for one day, but when that day stretches out into years, the strain can feel intolerable.

Some CFS sufferers do have occasional respites from their fatigue. For them, this symptom is intermittent rather than incessant. Others are completely bedridden. There is also a tendency for some people with this illness to feel different levels of fatigue at different times of the day. For instance, they may feel a little less tired in the morning. The only change I experience with this symptom is when it worsens, usually following activity.

I cope with my fatigue by acceding to its demands of rest, rest, and more rest. I don't like this new lifestyle that has been forced upon me, but I accept its stringent requirements because I have no other choice. This does not eliminate fatigue, but it does prevent me from feeling worse, and that is no small accomplishment. To someone with CFS, not feeling worse often seems like the next best thing to being cured. There is nothing that I do without first weighing the benefits against the detriments. I prioritize, eliminating from my schedule the activities that require the most amount of strength while giving the least reward, because I pay for every activity with the currency of exhaustion.

In the beginning, I was very resistant to this new lifestyle. I believed that letting CFS dictate my activities was tantamount to cowardly surrender. I thought that if I could be tough enough and persistent enough, I would conquer this illness. After years of making myself worse by foolishly trying to beat an unbeatable foe, I realized I was mistaking intelligence for cowardice. Mentally and emotionally I've neither given up nor given in. But, at least for now, I have surrendered to the absolute necessity of giving in physically. Only by resting do I have a chance of coping with this illness.

## MALAISE

When I'm grocery shopping I frequently have to sit down right in the middle of the store, not only because I am physically tired but because malaise makes simple mental tasks, such as choosing between two products, draining to the point of exhaustion. It can also make everyday tasks like phone calls seem complicated and overwhelming.

Malaise is my most devastating symptom. The word means "ill feeling," which to me is a terribly inadequate definition. How do I describe my worst nightmare? How can I be objective about something that I loathe? When I describe this symptom to people who have CFS, I call it "my sick, dazed feeling." They usually know immediately what I'm referring to. But that doesn't explain much to someone unfamiliar with CFS. If I said I was sick to my stomach, most people would understand exactly what I meant. But how do I tell you what it's like to be sick to my brain? I don't mean a headache; I mean a brainache!

When I feel malaise, my mind refuses to function properly, but it's not just an inability to think clearly. It's a pressure in my head that forces me to focus inward on my illness, making me unable to interact with the rest of humanity. It's as if a fence has been placed between me and the world, keeping it tantalizingly close, yet hopelessly out of reach. Even my senses are affected. Nothing tastes, feels, smells, sounds, or looks as good as it did before. My emotions can also be distorted. At times I feel completely emotionless, with none of the peaks or valleys of normal experience. Other times, just the negative emotions come through. My anger, frustration, and despair overwhelm me and I long to be back in the emotionless state.

The worst aspect of malaise is that it interferes with my ability to cope with my illness. How can I handle the tremendous burdens CFS imposes when malaise robs me of the emotional and mental tools I need to do exactly that? Though I feel like a prisoner of my own mind, I also feel surgically removed from it. In one sense I am locked in, but in another I am locked out.

There is another manifestation of this symptom called "post-exertional malaise." This is a sick, dazed feeling that affects your whole body after you have been active. Sometimes when I have pushed myself too hard, I am so overwhelmingly affected that I am too ill to perform even the simplest of tasks. It doesn't take hours to recover—it takes days.

Although I have not found any solutions to this dilemma, I have learned that there is a correlation between an increase in my activity and an increase in my malaise, so resting at least helps prevent a worsening of this symptom.

## SORE THROAT

A sore throat is another common symptom of CFS. While mine is painful, it is not constant and unrelenting the way my fatigue and malaise are. Another difference is that my malaise and fatigue don't become more severe until hours after an activity, while my sore throat gets worse almost immediately. It is one of the first indications that I have been pushing myself too hard.

This sore throat is not like those I experienced before I became ill. It is a much duller ache. While the pain can radiate all the way up to my ears and head, it seems to start much deeper down, in the throat. The pain and swelling may be centered near the vocal cords, too deep to be noticed by the average doctor using a tongue depressor. If your throat really hurts, you may want to go to an ear, nose, and throat (ENT) specialist. They have the proper instruments to examine your throat. Many times, only an ENT specialist will be able to notice any appreciable swelling or irritation.

The worst aspect of a sore throat is, obviously, that it hurts. Pain is not easily ignored. It seems to reach out and grab me and say, "Pay attention!" and I have no choice but to do just that. Unfortunately, I know of nothing to relieve the pain. Resting is preventive medicine, and gargling with warm salt water may bring temporary relief. Shawn, whose sore throat is constant and much more severe than mine, has discovered what she says is the only truly effective "treatment" for temporary (albeit fattening) relief of her sore throat: milk shakes. Her treatment may not be sanctioned by the medical profession, but it does seem to help. And besides, what other medicine can you look forward to taking with such pleasure?

## TENDER LYMPH NODES

Lymphadenopathy, the technical term for enlarged lymph nodes, is a common symptom of many diseases. But CFS patients tend to have a slightly different condition—tender lymph nodes without substantial enlargement. Lymph nodes are located throughout the body and function as a clearinghouse for the lymphatic system. This veinlike circulatory system collects the fluids, proteins, and foreign substances that accumulate between the cells of the body, and it recycles anything that can be reused.

Lymph nodes help to filter out and dispose of undesirable matter, such as bacteria or refuse. They are also the site where many of the white blood cells of the immune system are stored and matured. Therefore, enlarged or tender lymph nodes frequently indicate that the body is actively fighting an infection.

Even though lymph nodes are found throughout the body, your doctor will probably examine three main areas: the neck, under the arms, and the abdomen. While tender or enlarged lymph nodes are a normal and typically benign consequence of having certain infections, they should always be examined by a physician. Though it is not related to CFS, there are certain types of cancers, called lymphomas, that are associated with the lymphatic system. The effect of tender or enlarged lymph nodes is usually not serious, but can cause some pain and discomfort.

## UNREFRESHING SLEEP

In my opinion, this is one of the most devastating symptoms of CFS. For patients who crave sleep the way a starving man hungers for a morsel to eat, we are thwarted in our attempts to feel better by our lack of rejuvenating sleep. Studies have shown that even healthy people who experience the slightest sleep disruptions for the shortest of times become physically, mentally, emotionally, and psychologically impaired. CFS sufferers cannot expect to feel any differently. After all, many of us have been suffering from this harmful symptom for years.

It is not easy falling asleep when your throat hurts, your head is splitting, and your joints are aching. Thus, it is quite easy to understand that sleep, even for people as exhausted as we are, might not be easily achieved. But the inability to fall asleep is only part of what this symptom entails. Even if sleep finally does come, there is no guarantee that it will be long or restful. I have often slept soundly for twelve hours or more, only to wake up feeling as if I had hardly slept at all. And sometimes I wake up two or three times during the night, totally disoriented, which would affect anyone's sleep. Suffice it to say that anything you can do to improve this symptom would immeasurably impact your health for the better.

Many CFS patients find relief from low-dose tricyclic antidepressants, which help improve their sleep, and others try sleeping pills. I have been helped by taking a mild sedative for those nights when I hurt too much to fall asleep. Since sleeping pills can be addictive, I am very careful to minimize their use.

If you push yourself beyond your limits, allowing your body to rest only when you sleep, you should consider reevaluating your priorities and slowing down. The more you rest during the day, the less critical sleep will be at night.

## MEMORY LOSS

I personally find this symptom terribly disturbing (but I can't remember why!). I used to pride myself on my memory. In fact, it replaced diligent study as my principal means of getting through school. Now I have such a terrible memory that I sometimes don't even bother trying. Some people with CFS are affected more severely in their short-term memory—they can't remember where they just put something or what they are supposed to do the next hour. I have more difficulty with my long-term memory. For example, I have trouble remembering the names of people whom I have known for a long time.

Memory loss is another neurological symptom of CFS that may have a physiological component as well as a psychological one. Either way, I have unfortunately found nothing that helps alleviate this symptom. Shawn tries to write down lists of things she needs to remember. If she needs to remember something short term, like getting soap from the upstairs closet, she repeats "Soap" to herself until she finds it.

## HEADACHES

Headaches are miserable. Everybody hates a headache. What other relatively minor affliction is single-handedly capable of supporting its own multimillion-dollar-a-year drug industry? The problem is that you can't ignore a headache. It may be minor compared to other ailments, but it is major in its ability to prevent you from doing or thinking about anything else. You just can't be yourself until it is gone. This seems especially true of CFS headaches, maybe because they come in tandem with so many other horrible symptoms.

Fortunately, I don't have these headaches all the time. Like many other symptoms of this illness, my headache is worse when I have been active. Some people find relief with aspirin or other analgesics. I've tried most of the major pain relievers, but the only way I can relieve a headache is to turn out all the lights and lie down. Usually within a couple of hours the headache is gone.

## JOINT PAIN

As anyone confined to a wheelchair can attest, it isn't easy to be immobile in a mobile society. Our world isn't geared to accommodate those who can't keep up with its fast and frenzied pace. The joint pain that strikes many people with CFS can prevent them from doing just that.

Joint pain affects many different areas of the body, including the knees, ankles, fingers, wrists, elbows, shoulders, and hips. It varies in intensity and is not always constant. Some people are so debilitated they are actually confined to a wheelchair, others are able to get around by using a cane, and many are just not able to move as easily as they used to.

Many people notice that their joint pain is worse during a flare-up of their illness or following increased activity. For some, this symptom ebbs and flows for no apparent reason. In addition, joint pain associated with CFS occurs without any redness or swelling (making it another invisible symptom). Most people only experience this pain intermittently. During those times, they try to limit their activities, but if the pain strikes areas such as the arms or hands, simple tasks like cooking or cleaning can become a study in pain and frustration.

I consider myself quite fortunate because my experiences with severe joint pain have been infrequent. During particularly bad flare-ups of my illness, I may notice some pain in my knees. It isn't a sharp pain, more of a dull ache. However, during one flare-up I was driving in my car and the joint pain in my knee began to worsen every time I pushed the clutch down to shift. The pain got so intense that driving became impossible. When I got out of the car, I realized I was unable even to walk a few short steps. I went to see an orthopedist, but he didn't find anything physically wrong with my knees. He did fit me for braces, which enabled me to support myself with less pain and effort. After about four weeks the pain was suddenly gone. Not coincidentally, the relief coincided with the end of one of my CFS flare-ups. I haven't experienced such severe pain during any of my more recent flare-ups and I am not sure why. I am just thankful this symptom is not constant for me.

There seem to be a thousand times more questions than answers with this illness and even fewer methods of relief. For joint pain, you might try commercial pain relievers, similar to arthritis medications. If the pain becomes so severe that walking is difficult, ask your doctor for some prescription-strength medicine, and don't be embarrassed to use a cane or wheelchair.

## INABILITY TO THINK CLEARLY

At first glance, this must seem like a terribly unremarkable symptom and very similar to malaise. They are similar in that both affect the mind, but they don't always go hand in hand. In my experience, this symptom is different from malaise because it does not involve a sick, dazed, clouded feeling. Rather, it reflects confusion, impairing the ability to reason abstractly.

I am most aware of this symptom when I am attempting to concentrate. When reading, I will suddenly be unable to recall a single word I've just read. I can write a sentence and be unsure if what I've just written makes a bit of sense. And I can listen to people speak and not understand what they are saying. My wife is most affected by this symptom when she tries to drive. The roar of a passing truck, the changing traffic lights, the hubbub of pedestrians on the street all bewilder her, making the safe operation of a car very difficult. Even the simple act of crossing the street can be perplexing and mystifying.

The inability to think clearly can make a CFS patient appear slow or even mentally impaired. It is quite frustrating, especially for students who find themselves unable to complete their assignments or do well on tests, or those involved in business who can no longer keep up with their colleagues. Unfortunately, as with malaise, I have not found any relief for this symptom.

## MUSCLE PAIN

Generalized muscle pain or weakness has never been a symptom that I have suffered with to any great extent, but I do know quite a few people who have been devastated by it. I have a good friend who can't go anywhere without using a wheelchair or a cane. In fact, when he is hit by a weak spell it can be his most disabling symptom. Sometimes the weakness is localized in a particular area of his body, but many times it completely overwhelms him. While it seems that there is a loose correlation between activity and this symptom, I have seen him overcome by it for no obvious reason.

Shawn also experiences muscle weakness. She is only able to do physical tasks for a short time before she feels weak and needs to rest. Her arms and legs have a feeling of heaviness, which makes even simple tasks, like washing the dishes, an effort for her.

I know of other CFS sufferers who experience muscle pain more than weakness. Typically, it seems to be in the extremities and it too can be quite disabling. Some people also have horrible leg cramps. The only things I know of to relieve muscle pain are massage and medicines that act as muscle relaxers.

The symptoms described above are considered standards of CFS. By that I mean that they are the ones most frequently experienced. The symptoms that follow are not as universal. Some sufferers may experience them only once or twice and others not at all. Nevertheless, they are still important, they are simply not as common.

## FEVERISHNESS

Fever is one of the few symptoms of CFS that is objectively measurable, yet while many patients feel feverish, few will actually demonstrate a very high temperature. In fact, a high fever is not indicative of CFS and should be checked by a doctor. The entire time I have had CFS I have felt feverish, yet my temperature has rarely risen over 99° Fahrenheit. However, from a patient's perspective, a symptom is a subjective impression, not an objective fact. You need not have an inordinately high temperature to validate your feverish feeling.

I have not noticed any significant fluctuation in my feverishness during the course of a day. It never becomes very severe, but it also never goes away. There are people with CFS, however, who do feel more feverish depending on the time of day. Since this symptom is less severe than many of my others, it is difficult for me to discern exactly how it affects me. I know that it contributes to the flulike feeling that I associate with CFS, but it is not particularly devastating. I have not found anything that significantly alleviates this symptom beyond aspirin and cold compresses on the head.

## WEIGHT LOSS

Weight loss, while a symptom of CFS, has the distinction of being one of the few symptoms that does not appear to be directly caused by the illness. It may be that some people with CFS experience weight loss simply because they are too exhausted to prepare nutritious meals. Maybe their desire for food, like their desire for everything else, is suppressed by their illness. Perhaps they are so emotionally and physically depressed that they don't care enough about themselves to eat properly.

My only experience with weight loss came from trying "health-conscious" diets, every one of them guaranteed to make me healthy as an ox. All I did was lose weight that, being thin already, I could ill afford to lose. If you're interested in trying a diet, you might want to discuss it first with a nutritionist or your doctor.

If you find you are losing weight unaccountably, take a step back and try to determine the cause. If your desire for food is gone because nothing tastes good anymore, you have to begin regarding your food as you would medicine: It may not taste very good, but it is terribly important for your health.

## SKIN RASHES

I have experienced skin rashes only twice during my illness. The first time was when I went to see a doctor only a month after I became ill. Baffled by my early symptoms of fatigue and malaise, he didn't know what else to do for me and prescribed penicillin. Within a day, I had broken out into hives all over my body. I have since learned that hives are a classic reaction when someone with infectious mononucleosis is given penicillin.

The second time I had a skin rash was when I was a patient in an experimental drug therapy program at the National Institutes of Health. They were trying to determine the efficacy of acyclovir (an antiviral medication) on CFS. I broke out in welts, mostly on my abdomen. They were much larger but less numerous than the hives I previously had. In both cases, my rashes were in response to drug treatments. However, some people experience rashes even though they are not on any medication.

Since rashes are a common allergic reaction, it's possible that a patient's allergies are interacting with the illness. There does not seem to be one specific rash associated with CFS. Therefore, the illness may be unmasking preexisting allergic conditions that only now show themselves in the form of a rash. Ask your doctor or dermatologist for medication that can relieve this symptom.

## PERSONALITY CHANGES

Personality changes are practically synonymous with CFS. When I am feeling extremely ill, I have found that I feel like a different person. If I am not angry, I am sad. If I am not frustrated, I am depressed. I have so many negative emotions that I hardly remember what the old me was like.

What's happening is that my personality is reflecting whatever emotion I happen to be struggling with at the time. This illness has worn me down so completely that at times I have neither the strength nor the desire to put up façades. With only enough strength to survive one day at a time, there is no energy left over for masking my feelings, and occasionally other people see me struggle with these raw emotions.

This seems to me to be a natural consequence of living with such a taxing chronic illness. Beyond psychiatric intervention, should your mood swings get out of hand, I can only recommend that you help the people around you to understand what you are going through so they can be more patient and compassionate.

## IRRITABILITY

I had trouble deciding whether this symptom actually deserved a heading of its own. It could easily be included under personality changes and still be explained fairly well. I realized that this is such a common condition among patients with CFS that it merits special recognition.

Like my mood swings, irritability is dictated totally by my illness. Unfortunately, it is dictated often. I marvel at the times I am not irritable rather than at the times I am. Irritability is always just below the surface, ready to explode at any moment. Healthy people normally maintain a buffer zone that allows them to let life's little annoyances slide off their backs. But the frustration with my illness has gotten the better of my patience. I feel like a lion on the prowl, waiting for some poor unsuspecting person to say the wrong thing or, better yet, give me the wrong look. You know the look I mean, the one that tells you that no matter what they say, they really don't believe in your illness. When I feel better, I have more control over my emotions, and I say nothing. If I feel very ill, the person who commits so egregious an error receives the full brunt of my pent-up frustrations. Fortunately, I have found that the severity of this symptom has improved as my health has improved.

## NIGHT SWEATS

While night sweats are not as debilitating as most of the other symptoms, they are yet another peculiar piece in the CFS puzzle. I will sometimes suddenly awake to find myself dripping with perspiration, as if I had run a marathon in my sleep. Night sweats occur randomly and without warning, and so far I have been unable to identify the cause. Fortunately, they are nothing to be overly concerned about. Other than feeling uncomfortable, night sweats are quite painless.

## CHEST PAINS

I have never experienced this symptom, but any pain that might be associated with the heart should not be dismissed lightly. Some people with CFS experience a tightening around the chest. Some also experience palpitations, or a racing heart rate. Although there are no studies correlating CFS with this symptom, remember that you don't need to have CFS to have heart problems. You can have two totally unrelated ailments. So please go to your physician immediately when you experience any type of heart or chest pains. Don't dismiss chest pains simply because you have had them before or because you think they are merely another symptom of this syndrome. Chest pains always need further evaluation.

I have discussed the major and most common symptoms associated with CFS, but they are not the only ones. The following is a list of other symptoms that have been reported in the literature on CFS or that I have heard about from various CFS sufferers:

Depression
Dizziness
Disorientation
Odd skin sensations
Intolerance of temperature extremes
Swelling of the hands
Loss of muscle coordination
Weakness
Numbness and lack of feeling in parts of the body
Digestive problems
Intolerance of alcohol
Sensitivity to light and noise
Chills
Splenomegaly (enlarged spleen)
Hepatomegaly (enlarged liver)
Swelling of the eyelids
Nausea
Diarrhea
Tinnitus (ringing in the ears)
Earaches
Bladder problems
Excessive sleep or sleep disorders
Balance problems
Shortness of breath
Abdominal cramping

It is important to emphasize that not only enlarged lymph nodes or chest pains, but any serious symptom, should be reported to a doctor. CFS patients sometimes attribute everything they feel to CFS. This is potentially dangerous because we are still capable of developing other medical problems, mild or serious, that should not be ignored.

And finally, a discussion of CFS symptoms would not be complete if I didn't share an observation about the word *complaint*, which is often used in discussing symptoms. One of its dictionary definitions is "a bodily ailment or injury," which is how I mean it when I use it in reference to symptoms. But it's an easy word to misconstrue—and that makes it an interesting analog for my illness. Anyone who accepts the reality of CFS will understand what I mean by "complaint." A skeptic will hear it as a whine, a gripe. As with so much in illness, understanding rests in belief.

# CHAPTER THREE

# Diagnosis

*Chronic fatigue syndrome remains very much a "symptoms" disease. There are no blood tests or other laboratory methods to determine who is suffering from it. When making a diagnosis, doctors still must rely more on what a patient feels than on any objective evidence.*

Out of all the areas of CFS that I've written about in the past, I would have thought that the one to advance the most over the years would have been diagnosis. After all, how can we truly understand or even treat this disease without a definitive method to determine who has it? And yet, years later, we're still in the "dark ages" regarding the diagnosis of CFS. I presumed the increase in national attention would educate physicians, thereby making it easier for them to diagnose accurately patients who are experiencing prolonged fatigue. Unfortunately, this does not seem to be the case. Thanks largely to the tireless efforts of support groups and some wonderfully concerned physicians, some progress has been made, yet ignorance reigns supreme.

Just recently, I happened to overhear a woman telling her friend of her recent diagnosis of chronic fatigue syndrome. She didn't refer to any of the symptoms of CFS except fatigue, and her level of functioning had hardly been diminished. Yet her doctor, noticing slightly elevated results from a blood test for Epstein-Barr virus, had concluded that she was suffering from CFS. After all that has been done to instruct physicians about CFS, we still have doctors determining the diagnosis of a patient on the basis of one single test, a test that was long ago proven to be ineffective in the diagnosis of CFS. This woman may, in fact, have had a mild case of CFS, but it seems more likely that she was suffering from overexertion or some other condition. Unfortunately, until an accurate and reliable method for diagnosing CFS becomes a reality, our condition will rarely be thought of as anything more than pampered complaining of the overindulged. In short, it will continue to be known as the yuppie flu.

Not only does our inability to diagnose this syndrome interfere with patients receiving treatment for other maladies, but it also affects our credibility, both psychologically and socially. The burden of having an illness that still remains a wastebasket diagnosis—in other words if everything else has been ruled out, it's possible you have CFS—exacts a terrible toll. Most doctors, trained as scientists and therefore disinclined to believe what cannot be objectively verified, hesitate to rely on the subjective symptoms of their patients. And what doctors refuse to legitimize, society in general refuses to legitimize.

In fact, skepticism regarding the authenticity of our illness is one of the main reasons we have difficulty obtaining research grants for CFS. The powers that be are reluctant to finance research for an illness without an objective method of determining what that illness is and who has it. It is unfortunate that so much emphasis has been placed on the lack of a diagnostic test for CFS. Dr. Straus of the NIH points out that it is not unprecedented for researchers to commence study on diseases for which there are no definitive diagnostic tests; multiple sclerosis is just one example.

It has been my good fortune to be under the care of doctors who are not threatened by medical uncertainties or inexactitudes. They remind me of the old country doctors who knew that their patients were the best source of information when making a diagnosis. Some might argue that the doctors who practiced fifty or sixty years ago are an anachronism of a bygone era. They had no other choice but to listen to the musings of their patients because they did not have access to the modern-day technology that makes diagnosis less a subjective science and more an exact one. But I find it not merely coincidental that at the same time there has been an explosion in medical technology, there has been an equal explosion of dissatisfaction from patients treated by that technology.

Their dissatisfaction, it seems to me, stems from the fact that too few doctors are willing to listen to their patients. The old country doctors, usually responsible for their patients' total care, thoroughly knew each and every patient and were often called upon to dispense advice as much as medicine. But today many doctors have forgotten how to treat the whole person. Modern medicine examines a patient and sees a hundred different specialties. There is a doctor for feet, one for knees, one for skin, and even one for the brain, but there is rarely a doctor to care for the whole patient.

If you suspect that you have CFS, but have been unable to find a doctor who is knowledgeable about this syndrome, continue searching until you find one who is. Your doctor should be someone you can depend on for help, advice, and support. And when you do finally find a caring physician—and there are many wonderful ones out there—treat him or her with respect. Patients often vent their impatience and frustration on their doctors when medicine has little to offer in the way of treatments.

## ACHIEVING A DIAGNOSIS

Even though I've stated that symptoms are important in making a CFS diagnosis, I don't want any readers to decide they have CFS just because they feel sick and tired. Work with your doctor. The symptoms of CFS are general enough to be associated with a multitude of other illnesses, including many that require immediate attention.

# THE CRITERIA FOR DIAGNOSING CFS

Diagnosis of CFS is based on guidelines established by a group of internationally recognized researchers assembled by the Centers for Disease Control and Prevention. In the December 1994 *Annals of Internal Medicine,* these researchers, headed by Dr. Keiji Fukada, published a paper entitled "The Chronic Fatigue Syndrome: A Comprehensive Approach to Its Definition and Study." This case definition of CFS was established in order to ensure diagnostic uniformity of CFS patients for researchers and physicians. Treatments can be better evaluated as to their effectiveness when the patients studied have homogeneous symptoms. Since so much is still unknown about CFS, this definition is not set in stone. The researchers realized that many of the parameters they set may have to be changed as more is learned about this syndrome.

Your physician might want to read the paper in its entirety, but for patients I will summarize its findings. To put it simply, there are three major requirements you must satisfy before being diagnosed with CFS: You must meet the fatigue criteria, you must rule out other conditions, and you must present other accompanying symptoms.

## FATIGUE CRITERIA

1. You must have clinically evaluated, unexplained chronic fatigue, either persistent or intermittent, for a period of at least six consecutive months. This fatigue had to have a definite onset. You can't have suffered with it from the day you were born.
2. The fatigue cannot be the result of ongoing exertion, such as athletics, nor can it be significantly helped by rest. In other words, this eliminates the people who push themselves too hard or just need a vacation.
3. Your fatigue must be severe, causing you to reduce

significantly your activities associated with work, school, social or personal life.

## EXCLUSION OF OTHER CAUSES FOR CFS SYMPTOMS

Next, your doctor needs to be able to exclude your ailment from any other medical and psychological disorders, such as hypothyroidism or depression. This is achieved by performing complete exams, including blood and lab work, documenting a thorough history, and reviewing all medical records to define the factors present at the time of symptom onset. Any alternative explanation for your malady must be excluded. While not specifically mentioned in the case definition, some of the possible causes that need to be ruled out are as follows:

1. Chronic inflammatory disease (such as hepatitis)
2. Autoimmune disease (such as arthritis)
3. Neuromuscular disease (such as myasthenia gravis or multiple sclerosis)
4. Cancer (such as nasopharyngeal carcinoma, Burkitt's lymphoma, Hodgkin's disease, or other lymphomas)
5. AIDS
6. Fungal disease, bacterial disease (such as tuberculosis), and parasitic disease (such as toxoplasmosis)
7. Endocrine disease (such as diabetes or hypothyroidism)
8. Localized infection
9. Chronic psychiatric disease (such as endogenous depression, schizophrenia, or chronic use of major tranquilizers or antidepressive medications)
10. Drug dependency or abuse
11. Side effects of a long-term medication or toxic agent (such as a pesticide or heavy metal)
12. Other known or defined chronic pulmonary (lung), cardiac (heart), gastrointestinal (stomach and intestinal),

hepatic (liver), renal (kidney), or hematologic (blood) disease
13. Nonspecific illnesses such as environmental illness, Lyme disease, fibromyalgia, hypoglycemia, etc.

I realize this is an intimidatingly long list of diseases. This is because doctors want to ensure that patients are not misdiagnosed as having CFS when in fact they might have some other ailment. Check with your physician to determine which, if any, should concern you.

## OTHER SYMPTOMS

Finally, you must have four or more of the following symptoms. The only standard to be used is that these symptoms, persistent or relapsing, must also have occurred during the same six consecutive months of your fatigue.

1. Short-term memory loss or impaired concentration that causes substantial reduction in previous levels of your performance in school, work, social, or personal activities
2. Sore throat
3. Tender lymph nodes in the neck or axillary area
4. Muscle pain
5. Joint pain without swelling or redness
6. Headaches that are different in severity or type than any other headaches experienced before the onset of CFS
7. Nonrefreshing sleep
8. Post-exertional malaise. This is when you feel rotten for more than twenty-four hours after you have pushed yourself either mentally or physically.

It's important to remember that this working case definition was established to identify the typical CFS patient for research purposes. This was done to ensure that the many investigators studying this syndrome use patients who are comparable to those studied by other investigators. If you don't fit this definition, it doesn't mean that you aren't sick. It just means that you are suffering from something that cannot be clinically diagnosed as CFS for research purposes. If you have ruled out other causes, have extreme fatigue and at least a few of the other accompanying symptoms, then it is quite possible you have CFS. Until more is known about this illness and accurate diagnostic tests are developed, there will never be a foolproof method of determining who does and does not have this affliction. The researchers who wrote this case definition realize that with so much unknown about this syndrome, even their guidelines cannot be considered definitive.

## WHAT DOESN'T WORK

The following two tests are included in this chapter not because they are helpful in diagnosing CFS, but because they are not. There are still many physicians who are unaware of this fact and may still use these tests when determining your diagnosis.

### THE MONOSPOT TEST

Patients with CFS who can relate their illness to mononucleosis typically tell their doctors that their mono never went away; they know no other way to describe it. Typically, many of these patients are then given the standard monospot blood tests for mononucleosis. Unfortunately, this test does nothing to help diagnose CFS.

CFS is a completely different illness from mononucleosis, and too many doctors, unaware of this fact, wrongly assume that any result on the monospot test, either positive or negative,

determines the possibility of a chronic mononucleosis-like illness. While in the past CFS was linked to mononucleosis, it is
not now.


## THE EBV SEROLOGY TEST

In the mid 1980s, Epstein-Barr virus (EBV) was considered the
cause of this syndrome. Thus, this illness was referred to as
chronic Epstein-Barr virus (CEBV) before being renamed chronic fatigue syndrome. Therefore, many people were given the
EBV serology blood test. It measures the presence of antibodies
to the Epstein-Barr virus, from which the presence of the actual virus can be inferred. However, years ago most physicians
concluded that this blood test is not useful in diagnosing CFS.
There were several reasons for this conclusion. Not all patients
who do have CFS have abnormal test results, and there seems
to be no correlation between test results and the presence of
symptoms. In addition, many healthy individuals have abnormal EBV test results. EBV received such widespread attention
during the early years of research on this illness that, unfortunately, it frequently is the only thing doctors recall about CFS.
Therefore, though it shouldn't, to the uninformed it still remains
one of the primary factors in the consideration of a diagnosis of
this syndrome.

In some CFS patients, test abnormalities to EBV, while not
diagnostically significant, can be useful. They can, for example,
indicate a possible reactivation of the Epstein-Barr virus, or an
abnormal immune response.

Until sensitive and accurate diagnostic tests are developed,
diagnosis of CFS will remain difficult. Please remember that I
am not a doctor, and only a doctor can make or exclude a diagnosis of CFS. So find a doctor you can trust and work closely
with.

If you have been diagnosed with CFS, don't neglect to see your physician regularly and to have complete blood work done routinely. I can't stress strongly enough how important it is to check periodically for the presence of other infections or causes for your symptoms, as well as to monitor the state of your immune system. Even though most physicians are not yet able to determine the level of functioning of specific aspects of your immune system, they can gain a sense for the overall state of the system. This is important because not every symptom should be attributed to CFS. You deserve to be followed closely by a physician to differentiate what is caused by CFS and what may be caused by some other condition.

# CHAPTER FOUR

# Understanding Your Illness

*Only by understanding your illness can you gain the wisdom
you need to confidently take responsibility for your own health
and welfare.*

When I originally wrote that sentence, I was referring solely to
the scientifically identifiable aspects of the illness we label
chronic fatigue syndrome. Just as a scientist will tell you that salt
is a combination of sodium and chloride, I wanted to break CFS
down into its component parts. I wanted to enable readers to
understand their illness just as a mechanic understands an automobile. However, as I read that sentence now, I realize that the
truth of it goes far beyond this limited parameter. This illness is
not simply a medical mystery brought about by some immune-
system problem or infectious agent. It is only when it is examined in the context of our whole being—body, mind, soul, and
spirit—that CFS can truly be understood. I don't want this
chapter to be encyclopedic, full of mundane science with little
or no practical relevance. I want it to be inspirational, strength-
ening you to grab hold of your health and welfare and gain
some measure of control over the decisions that affect your
health. Only through knowledge do we gain the power to make
informed decisions about how to deal with this illness.

In addition, I have heard heartbreaking stories of people
who wandered from doctor to doctor, desperate to find someone to identify the cause of their suffering, or who suffered with
their symptoms because they mistakenly believed there was

nothing they could do to alleviate them. I want you to be armed with vital, objective information that you can use not only to validate the serious nature of your condition, but also to give you insight into how best to choose treatments.

The sad truth is, with an illness like CFS, whose history is so filled with confusion and doubt, gaining a clear understanding of what your illness is—and is not—is still very difficult. After all, many years have elapsed since I last wrote on this subject and, in some ways, it still seems like we are light-years away from comprehending CFS. Unfortunately, it may well be years, or even decades, before the true mysteries of this syndrome are unraveled. That is not to say that there aren't things we do know, as well as theories we can assume are plausible.

If you had an ailment that a doctor could remove surgically or cure with medications, you might be able to relinquish your responsibility for self-determination. But CFS is a perplexing syndrome that often takes doctors beyond their own knowledge and understanding, and into areas where they may be no more qualified than you to make decisions that will affect your life. Often a doctor will be able to offer you options—some potentially helpful therapy or treatment, perhaps even the chance to try an experimental drug—but will have no way of predicting the results, or even guaranteeing that you won't come to further harm. Only you can make a decision like that, and to do it intelligently you need to understand your illness first.

I am not suggesting you refuse the help of a loved one or that you spurn a competent doctor's advice. On the contrary, no other illness forces a person to rely more heavily on the help and support of others. But only you know the specific burdens you are dealing with; only you can decide how best to cope with those burdens.

This proposal may be frightening to some of you because it is much easier and less intimidating to leave the difficult decisions to someone else. But often what is easiest is not what is best. Because I try to learn all I can about my illness, I am in a position to work side by side with my doctors; they rely on me for information as much as I rely on them. Most importantly, never stop striving to learn more about your illness and the way it affects you. This book should provide a base, a starting point, toward a better understanding of CFS, but you should not limit your understanding only to what I have written. New and important information is constantly being discovered about illnesses in general and about CFS in particular. And I look to medical professionals to be my partners in trying to eliminate the various symptoms collectively referred to as CFS.

You may feel overwhelmed by the immense challenge of being fully responsible for your health. Please understand that what I am advising is a process, not an end unto itself. I am urging you to increase, slowly but surely, your understanding of this syndrome, and of how it specifically affects your life. As your understanding increases, so will your confidence.

I've tried to make the science in this chapter easy to understand, but some of you will probably find parts of it rough going. Don't worry. Read as much of each section as you can digest at one time. I've organized each section with the general, and most important, information first and the more technical material after. If you get stuck, go on to the next section, where you'll find more information that will be useful to you. Perhaps later, when you have a clearer picture of what the science is about, you will go back and fill in any pieces you've missed.

## CFS, MONO, AND ME

Like many people with chronic fatigue syndrome, I think of my illness as mononucleosis that never went away, the reason being that I'm unable to determine when my mononucleosis stopped and my CFS started. Unfortunately, many physicians also consider CFS to be mononucleosis that doesn't go away. That is because years ago this syndrome was linked to mononucleosis, and it received so much press that it left a lasting impression among some doctors. In their defense, the two illnesses can be so similar symptomatically that they may appear indistinguishable. In addition, some past episodes of similar fatigue syndromes have been referred to in medical literature as mononucleosis. In fact, one of the only early distinguishing characteristics between chronic fatigue syndrome and chronic mononucleosis was the duration of the disease: six months, to be exact. From my perspective, however, nothing terribly dramatic happened on the 183rd day of my illness; I felt just as miserable as I did the day before. Therefore, in recent years, doctors and patients have begun to recognize the importance of distinguishing between these two illnesses.

The primary reason for establishing a unique identity for CFS is to prevent the pain and frustration of a misdiagnosis. Since most CFS patients are unable to trace the onset of their illness to an initial episode of mononucleosis, these patients and their doctors might never consider the possibility that CFS was the cause of their symptoms.

The distinction between CFS and acute infectious mononucleosis is also crucial because, though a patient may not feel much of a difference between these two illnesses, they are quite different diseases. All too frequently, because a patient's blood test for acute infectious mononucleosis has come back negative, the patient's complaints are dismissed by a doctor who excludes the possibility of a chronic mononucleosis-like illness, such as CFS.

Nonetheless, I realize that the comparison of mononucleosis and CFS is inevitable, what with the symptoms, such as fatigue and malaise, being so similar. Even I still use the comparison at times when talking to people because it helps me to explain my unique and relatively misunderstood illness by likening it to one that is easier to recognize and understand.

## CFS AND EPSTEIN-BARR VIRUS

Many physicians used to believe that the principal infectious agent of CFS was the Epstein-Barr virus (EBV). In fact, this syndrome used to be referred to as chronic Epstein-Barr virus (CEBV). Today, however, researchers no longer believe that the EB virus has any relationship to this syndrome.

The reasons EBV is no longer considered a culprit are many, but two stand out: First, patients with this syndrome are just as likely to test positive for other conditions, such as cytomegalovirus, herpes simplex, or measles. Second, researchers no longer see a correlation between a positive blood test for EBV and the presence of CFS symptoms. The Epstein-Barr virus was originally thought to cause CFS because it was believed that most patients with CFS tested positive for the virus. It is now known, however, that normal, healthy individuals can have similar blood results to those of CFS patients, and that there are CFS patients whose blood tests reveal they have never even had EBV.

There is a true form of chronic Epstein-Barr virus, but it differs from CFS. It is a rare and severe illness with major organ involvement, and is typically accompanied by more serious conditions such as chronic hepatitis, pneumonia, anemia, and sometimes lymphoma. These patients have test results that demonstrate an exceedingly high presence of active EBV infection, much higher than in CFS patients.

Dr. Straus of the National Institutes of Health considers it possible that some CFS patients may be found to have a milder form of this chronic Epstein-Barr infection—especially those patients who lack certain antibodies to the EB virus, or those whose illness started as acute mononucleosis. The typical CFS patient, however, does not lack these antibodies, and the onset of CFS is usually correlated with illnesses other than mononucleosis, such as the flu or bronchitis. In others, symptoms develop more gradually, without an obvious link to any disease. The majority of CFS patients, therefore, are not believed to suffer from a chronic EB virus infection.

## CFS—CONTAGIOUS OR NOT?

While the exact cause of CFS is still unknown, the good news is that it does not appear to be contagious. Since both Shawn and I have CFS, it may seem odd for me to claim that we are no more infectious than the average person. But studies have shown that transmission of chronic fatigue syndrome between family members is unusual. To date, we know of only a few other married couples with CFS. The vast majority of spouses, siblings, relatives, or friends of CFS patients don't become ill. Shawn and I may have become infected from a common source. Even though the odds are against it, our doctors think we may both have immune incompetence toward this syndrome, or a genetic predisposition to become ill with CFS.

## VIRUSES AND THE IMMUNE SYSTEM

Even though the cause of CFS remains a mystery, many of the theories center around viral or immunologic origin. Therefore, before I deal with some of the possible causes of this syndrome, it will help to give you some information about viruses in general, as well as an overview of the human immune system.

Viruses are small organisms, about one-ten-thousandth the size of a pinhead, and are visible only through a powerful electron microscope. They are biologically simple organisms, consisting of an outer protein coat surrounding inner genetic material. Despite their simplicity, there is still much that is unknown about viruses and viral infections.

Patients, accustomed to being treated for bacterial infections with simple and effective medicines such as penicillin, always seem surprised to learn how little modern medicine can do to treat viral infections. While bacterial infections invade the organs of the body, viruses invade the actual cells. They invade the cells because, unlike bacteria, they are unable to reproduce on their own. They need to hijack the reproductive capability of body cells genetically in order to propagate. Since viruses live within the cells of the body, drugs that are able to destroy a virus may also destroy the cells that contain that virus.

Viruses infect the body in many different ways. Some are airborne; infection results from breathing air that contains the virus. Others, such as HIV, the virus associated with AIDS, are transmitted through the blood or by sexual contact. The EB virus, which causes mononucleosis, is typically spread through saliva, hence the nickname for mononucleosis is "the kissing disease of amorous adolescents." The EB virus can also be spread through blood transfusions and possibly through other forms of intimate contact.

Each type of virus has an affinity for a particular cell in the body. It is usually a cell that is biochemically susceptible to invasion by that virus. The EB virus attacks the B cells, one type of white blood cell that is part of the immune system. This disrupts the normal immune response.

After a virus invades the body, it touches down on a cell, much the same way a mosquito lands on your arm. It then enters that cell either by being absorbed directly across the cell membrane—the outer "skin" of the cell, as it were—or by puncturing the cell like a mosquito biting. Next, it releases its own genetic material into the cell.

Once inside, the virus quickly and effectively goes about the task of transforming an otherwise normal and healthy cell into a miniature virus factory. It reprograms the reproductive machinery of the cell to manufacture thousands of new viruses. What happens next depends on the type of virus as well as the type of cell infected. Some types of viruses, called lytic viruses, cause the host cell to burst open and die, unleashing a new gen-

eration of viruses to continue the struggle of invading and conquering.

Other viruses can cause a latent infection. These viruses are
capable of immortalizing the host cell. In other words, the host
cell still lives and reproduces, but with the virus inside it. The
genetic material of the virus remains stably present inside the
cell nucleus. When the cell divides, producing a new daughter
cell, the virus also divides, becoming part of every new daughter cell. This allows the virus to reproduce itself perpetually, as
long as the host cell lives. These viruses can create lifelong infections because, once inside the host cell, they can hide from
detection by the immune system. Other types of viruses leave
themselves vulnerable by bursting and destroying the very host
cell they need in order to survive.

Still other viruses can cause infections that persist and
reactivate. (Some doctors believe that this type of infection
could be involved in CFS.) The host cell is still preserved intact
as in latent infection, however, the virus is actively reproducing
itself. New viral particles are released into the body, causing an
increased and continuous immune response.

## THE IMMUNE SYSTEM RESPONDS

Within hours after a virus enters the body, the immune system
mobilizes for action. An incredibly complex sequence of separate yet interdependent events is set in motion, culminating in
the destruction of the invading virus. While the immune system
is still a perplexing and largely unexplored entity, enough is
known to give us remarkable insight into the body's amazing
ability to protect itself against infection.

The immune system has two basic functions: to recognize
anything that may be detrimental to your health, and to respond
protectively. This clever system not only protects against infections, but is also able to distinguish between self and nonself—

between what is you and what is not you—preventing the body's own cells from coming under attack by the immune system.

The immune system is able to recognize and respond to millions of different foreign intruders, referred to as antigens (an antigen being anything that triggers an immune response). The chief components of that response are called white blood cells. There are trillions of white blood cells in the body at any one time. The majority of them are stored in such areas as the spleen and lymph nodes, waiting to be called upon when needed. The relatively few that are circulating throughout the body act as sentinels, constantly on guard against anything that might do harm. There are many different classes of white blood cells. The most notable of these are divided into three groups, depending on the particular function they serve. These are the T cells, the B cells, and the macrophages.

## THE T CELL

When a virus invades the body it is the circulating T cells that recognize it as a foreign antigen. The surface of every infecting antigen is different from anything else found in the body. When a T cell comes into contact with this antigen, it calls for reinforcements by releasing chemical signals into the bloodstream. (These messages can also be released by other cells, such as macrophages.) Some of these chemical signals, called lymphokines (also called cytokines), have been isolated and identified, and may sound familiar. These include interferon and interleukin-I and -II. These chemical messages have many known and unknown functions. They regulate and communicate with cells of the immune system. They warn the body that there is an infection present, alerting the stored white blood cells that their help is needed. They also warn the cells in the infected area about the presence of the virus, causing the cells to become resistant to penetration by the virus. Lymphokines inhibit the reproducing capability of those cells, thereby inhibiting the reproductive capability of any virus that has managed to enter a cell. Conversely, lymphokines are also capable of stimulating the reproductive capability of cells of the immune system at the same time they are impairing the reproductive capability of viruses. They also initiate the inflammatory response, which is familiar to anyone who has ever cut a finger.

When the skin of a finger is cut, the body becomes vulnerable to the invasion of millions of bacteria and viruses. In order to prevent this infection from spreading, lymphokines, as well as a chemical named histamine, are released. These chemicals increase blood flow to the infected area by dilating the blood vessels, speeding up the deployment of the stored white blood cells. While blood flow is increased, the infected area is simultaneously sealed off from the rest of the body, thereby containing the infection and preventing it from spreading. The increase of blood flow, with the subsequent closing off of the infected area, causes the finger to become red and swollen.

Typically, any infection associated with a cut finger is mild enough to be contained within hours, and the damaged area heals within days. However, many infections are not so easily contained. If the infection is severe enough, it may actually make you ill. There is usually a lag time of approximately two days before the body has marshaled the full strength of the immune system to destroy the invaders. During that time, the virus has the upper hand, making you sick by destroying healthy and vital cells. The virus also acts like a parasite, siphoning the food and energy so desperately needed by the cells of the body.

Viral infections cause many symptoms, one of which is fever. Fever serves many purposes, but one of its main functions is suspected to be fighting the infection. Many viruses are unable to function effectively at higher temperatures. The elevation of body temperature, therefore, aids in the battle against infection.

Another common result of viral infections is loss of appetite. One possible reason for this is that blood flow is rerouted from low-priority areas, such as the stomach, to high-priority areas that contain the virus. This allows speedy deployment of white blood cells. This decrease in blood flow to the stomach may be experienced as a decrease in appetite.

The worst symptoms of viral infections are the feelings of sickness and fatigue. There are many theories concerning the cause of these symptoms. They may be caused by the release of certain lymphokines, which are known to produce many symptoms similar to CFS. The feelings of sickness and fatigue may be the result of the abnormal functioning of the immune system. Another theory is that these feelings may be caused by the effect of viruses on specific cell components. (Many researchers in Britain are concentrating their efforts on the effect of CFS on the mitochondria of the cell. The mitochondria act as the powerhouse of the cell to supply its energy.) Another theory focuses on the incredible amount of energy being used to fight this microscopic war. The size of the combatants may be small, but the drain of your strength and the strain on your body are not. The typical weapons used in this war are cellular toxins and poisons, called cytotoxins. These toxins are used by the immune system to kill viruses and bacteria, but because of their potency, they can also make you feel tired and ill.

T cells have more functions than merely recognizing antigens. They also serve as a type of on/off switch for the immune system. Certain T cells, referred to as helper T cells, stimulate the immune system to fight infection. Other T cells, referred to as suppressor T cells, switch off the immune system once the infection is under control. Certain T cells also have the capability of fighting infections directly. These specialized cells, called cytotoxic T cells, have the ability to destroy viruses directly by releasing cytotoxins. Another class of T cells, referred to as natural killer cells, are also able to attack a virus immediately and form the first line of defense against foreign invaders.

## THE B CELL

B cells, another type of blood cell of the immune system, are also required to fight infection and, like T cells, have many different functions.

The main function of B cells is to produce deadly proteins called antibodies. Antibodies are shaped like a Y and have very specific receptor sites on their surface, allowing them to recognize and attack one particular virus.

These antibodies fit into one particular virus the way a key fits into one particular lock. If the key is not engineered for that lock, it will not work. This specificity serves two purposes: It ensures that these powerful antibodies will attack only foreign antigens and not the cells of the body, and serves as a type of memory system, allowing the immune system to remember a specific infectious agent. When the infection is over, the immune system retains these specific antibodies. If that particular strain of virus should ever invade the body again, the immune system will be able to respond quickly and powerfully, preventing a recurrence of that illness.

The ability of the immune system to remember and recognize past infections is the reason vaccinations against certain diseases are effective. For example, when an injection of a severely weakened or dead form of the polio virus is given, the dead virus is not able to cause the disease, but the body still produces antibodies that remain in the system. In the future, should the body become infected with the live polio virus, the immune system will respond quickly to destroy the virus, preventing contraction of the actual disease.

To date, five classes of antibodies have been identified. These antibodies, also referred to as immunoglobulins, each serve a different function. Immunoglobulin M, known as IgM, is the largest of the antibodies. It is also the first antibody produced during an infection. After a few days, the smaller, faster, and more mobile antibody known as IgG takes over. IgG is by far the most numerous of all the antibodies, comprising over 70 percent of the antibody total. IgA is an antibody most frequently found in the nose and mouth. It serves as the first line of defense against airborne infections. IgE is the antibody implicated in allergic reactions, and little is known about the IgD antibody.

Unlike T cells, B cells do not have the capacity of attacking a virus directly. However, B cells produce a certain class of antibodies called neutralizing antibodies that can attack. B cells also produce another class of antibodies that, when combined with nine specialized proteins called complement proteins, can achieve this same effect. These proteins, which circulate throughout the blood, are lethal toxins that do not have the safeguard of specificity that antibodies do. They destroy any cell they come in contact with. A fail-safe system is necessary in order to handle these deadly proteins safely; B cells are that fail-safe system.

These nine complement proteins, when taken individually, are safe and harmless in the same way that charcoal, potassium nitrate, and sulfur are safe and harmless; it's only when mixed together that they become gunpowder. B cells are responsible for combining these proteins into a lethal concoction and holding that concoction to the virus to be destroyed.

Other classes of antibodies that are summoned to the infected area as reinforcements serve to incapacitate the virus, preventing it from entering the body's cells. They also attach themselves to the virus and serve as a recognition flag, or signal, enabling other, more lethal cells of the immune system to recognize the virus easily and destroy it.

As I have mentioned, B cells produce specific antibodies that destroy specific viruses. But one B cell would not be able to produce enough antibodies to handle thousands of viruses. It needs help. This help comes from a third type of white blood cell, called macrophages, which release a chemical called transfer factor. This is a message telling other B cells to employ the same specific killing capability as the first B cell. In other words, transfer factor stimulates other B cells to become identical clones of the first B cell. It "transfers" the genetic capability to fight a specific virus from one cell to another.

## MACROPHAGES

Macrophages, the largest of the white blood cells, have many other functions as well. One of the most important is phagocytosis. This means that these cells can destroy viruses by swallowing and engulfing them whole, kind of like an immunologic Pac-Man.

These scavengers are indispensable to the immune system because they not only engulf viruses, they engulf all the debris that has collected in the infected area. For, as in any war, the dead and debris of battle are strewn everywhere. There are poisons and toxins, as well as bits and pieces of the winners and the losers. If this decaying debris were not removed, the area would be no better than a toxic waste dump, poisoned and inhospitable to life. Macrophages remove all this toxic matter from the site of the infection, allowing it to heal and be restored.

# SOME POSSIBLE CAUSES OF CFS

At this point in our journey, there are far more questions than answers to the perplexing problem of understanding CFS. Most of what we have is speculation. For that reason, it is important to remember that what this next section describes are theories, not concrete facts.

### THE "NEW VIRAL STRAIN" THEORY

The new viral strain theory holds that people with CFS are infected with either a new or different strain of a known virus.

It is believed that there is something genetically different about this strain of virus that makes it particularly virulent and more difficult to destroy.

In fact, genetically different strains of viruses are not uncommon. This can be observed in the flu virus. Typically, the body immunizes against recurring illness by the same virus, yet people are susceptible to the flu every year. This is because the influenza are genetically different every year. The body builds immunity to one strain one year, but fails to recognize the new strain the next. I realize that this makes viruses seem almost intelligent, but they are no different from any other organism. In order to survive, they are constantly adapting to suit their environment better.

Therefore, CFS patients may, in fact, have encountered a different strain of virus than what is typically found. Whether this different strain is particularly stronger or is just not easily recognized, it is overwhelming the immune system. Even if this theory were true, however, it still does not explain our inability to recover from this infection. With the flu virus, though the body may be unable to recognize each new strain immediately, in the end the immune system does prevail. Not so, it seems, with CFS.

## THE "RECURRENT VIRAL" THEORY

This theory holds that there is a reactivation of a virus that the body had previously beaten into submission. For example, at one time or another, most everyone is exposed to Epstein-Barr virus (EBV), a member of the herpes family of viruses such as herpes simplex, which causes cold sores. In fact, infection with this virus is so common that 90 percent of the adult population of the United States over age thirty has been infected with EBV. Most people who have recovered from an initial infection have no symptoms from then on. This is because with most herpesviruses, the body typically develops immunity against further outbreaks of the disease associated with that virus. In other words, the virus is still present in the body, but in a latent and inactive form. Despite that immunity, however, it can happen that the disease associated with a latent herpesvirus recurs. For example, some people continue to have outbreaks of oral or genital herpes. One suggested reason for this is that some people's immunity may not be adequate to prevent symptomatic recurrences. It is therefore theorized that patients with CFS may be experiencing a reactivation of a viral infection due to some environmental stress or genetic susceptibility affecting their immune system.

It is also possible that there could be a combination of the new strain and recurrent viral theories. Two or more viruses, a new strain, or a reactivated virus may act synergistically, flourishing together where neither would flourish alone.

## THE HORMONAL DEFICIENCIES THEORY

It is theorized that in some CFS patients, the body's ability to regulate the production of hormones by the endocrine system may be disrupted. (The endocrine system is comprised of glands, like the adrenal glands, which among other things are responsible for metabolism—the conversion of food into energy.)

When the body responds to physical or psychological stressors, the endocrine, or hormone, system reacts. A chain reaction is started by an area at the base of the brain called the hypothalamus. It releases a brain chemical called corticotropin releasing hormone (CRH), which causes the pituitary gland to release adrenocorticotropin hormone (ACTH). And finally, ACTH causes the adrenal gland to produce cortisol.

Research findings on the endocrine system from the National Institutes of Health reveal two hormonal deficiencies in CFS patients: There is a CRH deficiency, and this deficiency affects the hormonal pathway, resulting in a cortisol deficiency as well. These findings are very interesting because they offer a possible explanation for some of the symptoms of CFS. For example, low levels of either CRH or cortisol could cause insufficient stimulation of certain parts of the brain, resulting in fatigue, lethargy, and an increased need for sleep, all hallmarks of CFS.

Low cortisol levels may also affect the immune system. Dr. Straus of the NIH says, "Because cortisol is a potent suppressor of immune responses, a mild reduction in cortisol levels could allow the immune system to remain overactive, leading to findings such as higher-than-normal antibody levels to viruses in CFS patients."

These hormonal deficiencies may also offer a possible explanation for the depressive symptoms that can accompany CFS. It has long been known that the body's reaction to hormone imbalances can cause depression. In CFS, therefore, there might be a defect in the central nervous system that causes this biochemical imbalance, resulting in depression. This is not to say that CFS is being equated with depression, for people with classic melancholic depression have high cortisol levels, while CFS patients have low levels. However, it is possible that the depression related to, or caused by, CFS may trace its root to a physical defect in the endocrine system. Further studies are being completed at the NIH to determine whether treatment with small amounts of cortisol would improve hormonal imbalance and relieve any symptoms for CFS patients. There is also ongoing research into the effect of viral illnesses on hormone pathways.

## IMMUNE-DYSFUNCTION THEORIES

Some researchers believe that CFS patients have some sort of immune dysfunction. Some crucial link in the immunologic chain of events is defective, missing, or altered. From reading even my simplified overview of the immune system, you can see that it is a very complex system. There are literally hundreds of different ways the immune system might be defective. The body needs every part of the immune system to function cohesively and properly in order to control infection. Each individual part is vital to the whole. CFS patients may have too few or too many suppressor T cells, or deficient IgG antibodies. The inflammatory control may be lost or T cell recognition may be blocked. Maybe the immune system was depressed when an infection was first contracted, and it hasn't been able to recover since.

Researchers at the NIH have reported finding immune abnormalities in CFS patients—they have significant differences in the number and character of CD4+ T cells compared to healthy individuals. These cells are very specific, becoming linked to one type of invader, acting like traffic cops, directing the mobilization of the rest of the immune system.

CFS patients have a slight decrease in CD4+ T cells. In AIDS, these cells are destroyed, whereas in CFS they seem to be shifting location from the blood into the tissues. This is important for two reasons, one being that it explains why these cells are not detected in blood tests. The other is that when CD4+ T cells are in the tissues they release molecules to regulate the immune response, which can cause pain and inflammation. While these subtle abnormalities do not necessarily reveal the cause of CFS, they may explain some of its symptoms, such as muscle and joint pain and tender lymph nodes. People with inflammatory bowel disease experience pain in their intestines due to the same process. The reason behind the shifting of these cells is not yet known, but it may be caused by exposure to an infectious agent, or underlying neuroendocrine or neuropsychiatric abnormalities.

Some patients have other immune abnormalities, such as a deficiency in one of the subclasses of IgG antibodies (see the section on gamma globulin in Chapter 5, "Treatments"). Other patients exhibit a higher number of circulating immune complexes (an immune complex is the joining of an antibody to an antigen). Some patients have abnormal ratios of helper T cells to suppressor T cells. And still other patients exhibit suppressed activity of unique classes of cytotoxic white blood cells such as neutralizing antibodies and natural killer cells.

Other possible immune dysfunction theories include the theory that sustained activation of the immune system may cause CFS symptoms to persist, even though the original causative agent, such as a virus, is no longer active. In other words, there may be some dysfunction that does not allow the immune system to relax. It is possible that, like a car engine that will not shut off, the immune system is overreacting, wearing us out, because it is not recognizing that the infection has been brought under control.

Another possible result of an overactive immune system is the production of antibodies to different viruses. Because of this, we must be wary of assuming that whenever a CFS patient demonstrates the presence of a virus, like EBV or HHV6 (human herpesvirus-6), the cause of the syndrome has been discovered. In fact, the presence of a virus may be more indicative of an immune abnormality. The virus may not be the cause of our syndrome, it may just be taking advantage of a dysfunctional immune system. This could explain why some CFS patients have been shown to respond positively to tests for different viruses or diseases, such as EBV, CMV (cytomegalovirus), herpes simplex, and measles.

Perhaps the immune system is overproducing lymphokines, such as interferon or interleukin, or is producing them long after the initial infection has been resolved. These lymphokines are used to fight infection and regulate the immune system, and are thought to produce many of the symptoms associated with CFS, such as fatigue, feverishness, malaise, muscle aches, and depression.

It is interesting to note that lymphokines are not released during every type of infection. For example, they are not released during infection with German measles or the common cold, illnesses that do not share the flulike symptoms of CFS. And yet, in infections that are known to precede the onset of CFS, such as the flu or mononucleosis, lymphokines are produced.

Another theory postulates that there might be a genetic defect in the immune system. People with CFS may have inherited an inability to fight this syndrome in the same way others inherit sickle-cell anemia or Down's syndrome. There may also be genetic signals that keep individual viruses dormant. If latent viruses are involved in causing CFS, there may be a defect in the molecular on/off switch that controls these infections.

## THE ALLERGY THEORY

This immune-related theory suggests that patients with CFS may have an allergic hypersensitivity that has somehow become unmasked. As many as 80 percent of CFS patients do have a history of allergies, compared to 15 percent of the general population. When an allergic reaction occurs, the IgE antibody binds to the allergen (the foreign substance that induces the allergy), causing a release of histamine. Histamine is responsible for many of the symptoms related to allergy, such as fatigue, headaches, respiratory problems, and so on. Since such a high percentage of CFS patients have allergies, it may be possible that their immune systems are overreacting to the presence of general infectious agents in the same way they overreact to the presence of allergens.

Whatever the mechanism, the common thread in all these theories is that some part of the immune system is being either inhibited or overworked. It may even be too simple to suppose that the cause of CFS is that the immune system is either overactive or underactive. It is possible that CFS may be caused by a combination of the two. In fact, current data indicate that in some CFS patients, some immune functions are overactive while others are normal or underactive. The overall functioning of the immune system is still intact, which explains our ability to fight off other infections, but some vital immunologic response, critical to the control of whatever causes CFS, may be missing.

As with viral theories, we must also exercise caution in regard to immune-related theories. After all, it is difficult to determine whether immune abnormalities could cause CFS or could be a result of the disease process itself.

## NEUROPSYCHOLOGICAL INVOLVEMENT

There is still considerable debate regarding the role that neuropsychological factors play in CFS. In any illness, there is information that prevents us from completely disregarding this possibility, for clearly there is a link between the psyche and the immune system. As an example, patients who are depressed have been shown to be immunologically different from nondepressed patients. In addition, stress and depression can have a dramatic effect on the body's ability to recover from infection.

While there is evidence that depression, or other neuropsychological factors, can affect us physically and immunologically, there is no evidence that these factors cause CFS. Researchers have discovered too many physical, immunologic, and hormonal dysfunctions to warrant any other conclusion.

## NEURALLY MEDIATED HYPOTENSION (NMH)

Neurally mediated hypotension (NMH) is a condition that typically manifests itself in the form of dizziness and light-headedness. It is caused by a defect in the autonomic nervous system, which controls heart rate and blood pressure. Normally, when you have been sitting for a while your blood tends to pool in your legs due to the force of gravity. When you stand up, the blood needs to be redistributed. Your heart typically responds by increasing blood pressure and heart rate. Unfortunately, in people with this condition the heart slows down and blood pressure decreases. Just at a time when you need increased blood flow, your body shuts it down, causing light-headedness and fatigue.

This blood pressure condition offers a possible explanation for some of the symptoms of CFS, such as exhaustion, exercise intolerance, muddled thinking, difficulty concentrating, and dizziness. In the March 1995 issue of *The Lancet,* Rowe, et al. described this condition as a possible cause for CFS. He tested CFS patients for neurally mediated hypotension using a tilt table, because the condition can't be detected by standard blood pressure tests. Patients were gradually taken from a horizontal position to a vertical one, all the while measuring their circulatory response to the increased stress. Patients who were so diagnosed reportedly responded very well to treatment for this condition.

Perhaps a subset of CFS patients have been misdiagnosed with CFS and have been suffering from hypotension all along, or perhaps CFS contributes to the development of hypotension. For example, it is known that prolonged inactivity causes deconditioning, which contributes to the problem of blood pooling in the extremities. This may be why some CFS patients develop NMH.

It certainly seems plausible that patients with this condition could see an improvement in some, though probably not all, of their symptoms with treatment. Fortunately, many facilities, including Johns Hopkins Medical Center and the NIH, are researching the prevalence of neurally mediated hypotension in CFS patients, as well as their response to different treatments for this condition.

## NERVOUS SYSTEM ABNORMALITIES

Some physicians believe that CFS is caused by a defect in the central nervous system, such as the brain or spinal cord. This is because so many CFS symptoms seem to be neurological in nature, like memory loss, an inability to think clearly, and sleep problems. Some doctors find clues of this possibility in abnormal MRIs of the brain, but other doctors have not been able to confirm these findings. Some doctors are researching biofeedback techniques, and one has seen improvement in patients after performing surgery to correct a purported decompression of the spinal cord in the neck region.

With so many theories to choose from, who can predict which—if any—will turn out to be the cause of CFS? Perhaps several of these theories, as opposed to only one, may be correct. It is my opinion that researchers will one day discover that CFS is not really one specific illness, but rather a broad classification encompassing many different subclasses. These subclasses will be similar symptomatically, but will probably have different causes. In other words, although CFS patients share the same symptoms, the reasons why they are sick will be found to be different.

While this theory is just my opinion, there are plenty of precedents for it. Diabetes, for example, is divided into more than one type. Diabetics have an insulin problem; they are not able to break down blood sugar, the basic energy source for the body. Some diabetics are unable to produce insulin in their pancreas and are treated with insulin injections. Others are able to produce the insulin but are unable to utilize it. These people are usually treated with diet and exercise.

Similarly, we may all share a common syndrome referred to as CFS. We may have a common history and common symptoms as well. We may even share the same infectious agent. But the reasons that each of us is chronically ill may be different, and therefore different treatments would be required. There are countless theories for the cause of CFS. Right now, any or all of them may be right. It will be interesting to discover which, if any, most closely explains the cause of CFS.

# Treatments

*A waiting game! This illness has turned my life into a waiting
game. Rather than revel in the joy of a healthy and happy life,
I am forced to sit idly by with subdued anticipation in the hope
that someone, somehow, somewhere will discover a cure for
chronic fatigue syndrome.*

If someone were to ask me what is the most significant thing he
or she can do to recover from chronic fatigue syndrome, my
answer would be a simple one: Stop trying to cure CFS, and
start trying to alleviate your symptoms. Since I first became ill,
there have been dozens of promising cures for CFS just waiting
to be tried. I took suggestions from most any source, from my
doctor to my next-door neighbor. I tried everything, from aloe
to Zovirax, confident that at least one of them would make me
well. But as the years went by, I slowly exhausted the list and
still did not find a cure for my illness. It wasn't until I started
looking at each symptom independently, rather than at the illness as a collective whole defined as CFS, that I began to find
treatments that made me feel better. In other words, I went from
searching for "the" cure to seeking out numerous "mini-cures"
to help alleviate some of the pain and sickness.

Even though there is no known cure for CFS, this does not
mean I have given up my dream of one day being totally well
again. However, I realize now that discovering the means to that
end is best left to other sources. We have many wonderful
health and research organizations, national and local support

groups, and individual physicians working tirelessly for just such a cure. On the horizon there are always new medications and therapies being discovered that may someday lead to a cure.

And, this is not to say that people with CFS don't get well. On the contrary, there are quite a few who have. Some recovered spontaneously, while others attribute their restored health to some of the treatments discussed in this chapter. Most, however, like me, have only achieved partial relief through some of these treatments, and that is why this chapter focuses on symptom relief.

I am sure that all of us have, in our own minds, a minimum standard of health we need in order to have some semblance of a normal life. For me, being completely well remains a distant dream, yet some measure of improved health now seems achievable. As of now, it is this "middle ground," which lies between good health and total disability, that seems to be the best that most people with CFS can hope for. If truth be told, it is an area that I would dread existing in if I were totally well, and yet since I am still disabled, I aspire to it. It is a uniquely individual place, where fatigue is more a hindrance than a holocaust, and pain is more a distress than a disability. It is no small thing to hope for an improvement where CFS no longer controls you, but instead you obtain some measure of control over CFS.

Therefore, when trying treatments, I no longer use the more demanding criterion, "Will it make me well?" Instead, I ask myself, "Will it make me feel even the slightest bit better?" By reducing my expectations of the various therapies I try, I find myself more encouraged than discouraged by their effect. In order for a treatment to be effective as a cure it needs to be close to 100 percent beneficial, but now I am willing to settle for even a 5 percent improvement in my health.

Achieving a modest benefit of 5 percent when you are still 95 percent disabled may not seem like much. In fact, when you feel so sick it may be difficult even to notice such a minor change. But if you can find six different treatments that each gives you a 5 percent improvement, before you know it you are feeling almost one-third better!

Now I realize that this approach doesn't make for very good science. The argument could be made that by combining so many different therapies over a long period of time you really won't be able to distinguish properly which therapies are doing the most good. While that is true, to be perfectly honest I no longer care. I only care about feeling better, and trying different combinations of treatments is the only thing that has improved my health in the slightest. The important thing is to work closely with your doctor to avoid any possibly dangerous interactions or harmful side effects.

The inspiration for this new mind-set came from watching a magazine show a few years ago, featuring the mother of a little girl with Down's syndrome. Undaunted by the lack of treatments offered by the medical community, she took it upon herself to help her daughter. She spent years trying different combinations of vitamins, herbs, diet, and pharmaceuticals, and the results she achieved were nothing short of remarkable. Her daughter improved in just about every area of her life, even the way she looked. It wasn't a cure, but the impact on her daughter's life was incredible nonetheless. Therefore, though I always research treatments first in order to minimize any risk to my health, I now believe that I may never be able to feel better if I am not willing to experiment. To me, it is no different from when I went to the NIH to take part in their research for acyclovir, an antiviral medication. The key is to be monitored and followed closely by medical professionals who can give you the information you need to proceed safely with your treatments.

You may have read the story of the physician from New Zealand who tried to convince the medical and pharmaceutical communities that ulcers were bacterial infections and could be treated effectively with antibiotics. Obviously, with billions of dollars and hundreds of reputations at stake, he was denounced as a quack. He persevered, though, and eventually proved his point, but not before thousands of ulcer patients suffered more than they needed to. What I am trying to say is that while modern medicine is more often than not quite beneficial, it does not always hold the answers for all medical conditions.

If we aren't open to new therapies and ideas, who will be? Some people won't try a treatment unless it has been proven in a double-blind placebo-controlled study. While that is the preferred method, I don't want to wait that long. I know we all run the risk of trying inadequate and expensive treatments, and sometimes we run the greater risk of actually harming ourselves. But with proper care, monitoring by physicians, communication with other CFS sufferers, and common sense, I truly believe we can minimize those risks to an acceptable level.

I realize that reading that there is no cure may come as a shock to some of you. I remember being told that I would just have to learn to live with my illness. I had no intention of learning to live with it! I was sure it was only a matter of time until I found a cure. When reality finally did sink in, so did depression and despair: My disease was incurable. Especially for those of you who are new to CFS, I may have painted a gloomy picture, but take heart; our plight is not being ignored. The growing public awareness of our illness is sparking an increase in research funding. We also have many dedicated doctors who are striving to understand and treat CFS. Not a day goes by without some increase in our ability to heal fellow members of the human race. We will benefit immensely from these advances, even if they are not directed specifically toward CFS. The increased attention focused on diseases ranging from herpes to AIDS can only help further our cause. As scientists unravel the secrets surrounding viruses, the immune system, the neuroendocrine system, DNA, etc., they may also unravel the secrets surrounding CFS. So don't be discouraged! I truly believe it is only a matter of time until a cure for CFS is achieved, and, until that time, you may be able to significantly improve many of your symptoms using the therapies I describe in this chapter.

There are some important points I wish to emphasize before I begin discussing treatments. As addressed in Chapter 4, "Understanding Your Illness," the causes of CFS may differ from person to person. Therefore, the efficacy of a particular treatment should not be dismissed simply because you heard, through the grapevine, that it did not help someone else. As long as the treatment is safe, has a fairly good chance of making you better, and is approved by a competent physician, it is worth a try. Evaluate each and every potential therapy objectively; decide with your head, not with your heart. And be wary of anyone who seems more interested in your money than in your health. I have spent thousands of dollars chasing after worthless treatments because I was desperate to try anything to get well.

More than likely, you are trying different treatments or may do so in the near future. I have a recommendation: Familiarize yourself with the *Physicians' Desk Reference* (PDR). It is an important reference book used by doctors to obtain information about medications. It lists recommended dosages, possible side effects, and contraindications (circumstances when you should not use that drug). The PDR can help you make informed decisions regarding medications you might try. Your local library or your physician should have one. Don't be intimidated by the long lists of side effects; the PDR is required to list them all, no matter how unlikely or rare. Discuss them with your doctor to determine which side effects should concern you.

You may also want to contact the pharmaceutical company that makes the medication you are considering. Either a pharmacist or the *Physicians' Desk Reference* can tell you which company makes a particular medication. Shawn and I did this with a number of the medications we tried because we wanted to learn all we could about them. The pharmaceutical companies should be aware of possible risks as well as the proper use of their drugs. They are also aware of current research into the efficacy of their drugs in treating various illnesses. When we inquired, they were very helpful and were willing to answer any questions we had. Between your doctor, the PDR, a pharmacist, and the drug companies, you should be able to make wise decisions regarding any possible treatments.

When discussing treatments with your doctor, you should be actively involved in every decision. There are too many physicians willing to tell patients anything and everything they want to hear—some do so to placate, but others merely to profit. Either way, there is a price to be paid, to your finances or your vitality. This was never much of a problem in the early years of this syndrome. Back then you couldn't get anyone to listen to you, let alone claim any success with treatments. Years ago we suffered from physicians who didn't believe, but rarely from ones who couldn't be trusted. Now that CFS has become a national obsession, there are myriads of people out to exploit it for their own purposes.

Finally, the treatment recommendations for CFS change so rapidly and vary so much from doctor to doctor that I found it impossible to discuss all the treatments I have known people to try. In response to the first edition of this book, I received hundreds of letters from CFS sufferers, kindly offering treatment suggestions they had found particularly effective. One person recovered by eating nothing but asparagus, raw potato peels, red delicious apples, and salad with olive oil. I tried this diet with no success, but a better understanding of why so many people hate asparagus. Another person was physically attacked, suspended upside down from a ninth floor balcony, and literally "scared" well.

Even the treatments suggested by physicians may, at first blush, seem no less unusual. There are doctors prescribing nitroglycerin, the medicine used for heart patients. Others are performing brain surgery. The point is, a book can never keep up with the rapidly changing world of CFS treatments. Since I am not a doctor, I can only share my personal experiences, from one CFS patient to another. Therefore, I am only going to speak to those treatments I have tried, or am thinking of trying, with special emphasis given to those Shawn or I have found effective.

## KUTAPRESSIN

Though we can never discount the possibility of placebo effect, having both Shawn and me ill gives us twice the opportunity to test a medicine's effectiveness. Of the dozens of therapies we have tried, this is one of the only medications that have made a significant difference in both our lives. The chief benefit we received from kutapressin is that both Shawn and I feel stronger, with less weakness. This enabled us to begin exercising for the first time, which I believe increased our energy levels. In addition, Shawn saw a difference in her cognitive ability, and began reading books for the first time in many years. And our greatest improvement, which we thank God for every day, is that we no longer suffer that toxic, "poisoned" feeling to the same degree. It is not totally gone, but it is very much improved.

Kutapressin is a porcine (from pigs) liver extract composed of peptides and amino acids, which are organic compounds forming some of the building blocks of life. It has been in use since the 1940s, most commonly to control inflammatory reactions for skin disorders. If, as some postulate, our condition stems from a hyperactive immune system, it is believed kutapressin has a modulating effect. It has few side effects but, since it is extracted from pigs, an allergic sensitivity to pork should always be considered before administering this medicine. In addition, kutapressin should not be taken with MAO inhibitors.

While many physicians are using this medicine, we followed the protocol established by Drs. Steinbach and Hermann from Houston, Texas. They have had considerable experience administering this drug to hundreds of CFS patients, and claim to have incredible success with it. Kutapressin comes in liquid form and must be injected into the muscle, a daunting task for most of us unfamiliar with such a procedure. But most people, when working with a doctor, are able to learn how to administer it.

Therapy with kutapressin typically starts with an injection every day for a month. After that, the regimen is slowly decreased to three times a week over the next two months. It was at this point that Shawn's and my reactions began to diverge. I was eventually able to maintain my improvement while taking injections three times a week, but Shawn was not. She needed it more frequently than that to maintain her improvement. Some CFS patients are able to decrease the use of this medicine slowly until they are off it completely with no deleterious effects. Others need to maintain their injections for a much longer period of time.

One month I began doling out smaller doses because we were running out of medicine. Since I administer Shawn's injections as well as my own, she was unaware of what I was doing. Even after we obtained more medicine I continued with the lower dose, without telling her, to see if it would make any difference. Not only did she relapse, but when she found out what I had been doing, I was in big trouble. I learned two valuable lessons from this experiment: First, kutapressin does indeed seem to help alleviate our symptoms. And second, you should never use your wife as a guinea pig without her permission.

Some people use vitamin B-12 injections along with kutapressin for a supposedly enhanced effect, but neither Shawn nor I noticed any significant difference. The only drawback we experienced with this medicine is that it hurts, both physically and financially. Kutapressin is very expensive, between $85 and $115 a vial, with each vial containing 10 injections. In addition, it is injected into the muscle, typically the upper quadrants of the buttocks, so it can be a bit painful. I guarantee, though, that if you begin to feel any improvement, you will gladly tolerate the momentary pain for the lasting benefit. Kutapressin has made a bigger impact on our illness than anything we have ever tried. That does not mean it is a miracle drug that will eradicate CFS, but it seems to be quite effective in relieving some symptoms in some patients.

# ANTIDEPRESSANTS

There are three types of antidepressants used for treating chronic fatigue syndrome: tricyclic, MAO inhibitors, and serotonin reuptake inhibitors (SRIs). I will discuss each type in relation to its use for treating CFS.

## TRICYCLIC ANTIDEPRESSANTS

Tricyclic antidepressants have traditionally been used by doctors to help alleviate depression, but they are used in treating many other illnesses as well. This type of antidepressant, such as Sinequan or Elavil, is one of the most successful and highly recommended treatments for chronic fatigue syndrome. In fact, many CFS patients have experienced significant relief from fatigue and some of the neurological symptoms associated with CFS.

While the exact reason they are effective is still unknown, it is believed that they either help in the achievement of restorative sleep or have some sort of modulating effect on the immune system. When they are used for treating CFS, they are administered in very low doses, much lower than that used for depression. Therefore, in this application, the name antidepressant is misleading.

I have tried many tricyclic antidepressants with little improvement. Shawn, however, did experience some improvement while on an antidepressant called Pamelor. Her throat and glands were less swollen and painful, her energy level slightly improved, and the malaise lessened.

In low doses, short-term use of tricyclic antidepressants is considered safe, but they can have serious side effects (especially with long-term use) and need to be prescribed and followed by a physician experienced in their use. The only side effects I experienced were merely unpleasant: a dry mouth, weight gain, and mild insomnia. Shawn, however, also experienced abdominal cramps, mild chest pains, and a racing heartbeat until her body adjusted to the medication. If one tricyclic doesn't relieve some of your symptoms, it is possible that another one will.

## MAO INHIBITORS

Another class of antidepressants, called MAO inhibitors, inhibit an enzyme called monoamine oxidase. MAO is found in the mitochondria of certain cells (the mitochondria act as the powerhouse of the cell). While the therapeutic effect of MAO inhibitors, such as Nardil or Parnate, for CFS is still anecdotal, enough interest has been raised so that scientific studies are being undertaken.

The most serious drawback of MAO inhibitors is the possibility of dangerous side effects. You can experience a dramatic increase in blood pressure or an exceptionally high fever if you mistakenly combine these drugs with certain medicines, foods, or beverages. These are very dangerous situations, and in extreme cases could be fatal. Therefore, the use of these drugs requires strict supervision by a physician, as well as certain dietary restrictions—you need to be aware and well informed. Any substances that contain a high tyramine content must be avoided. These include, but are not limited to, aged foods such as cheese or wine. You also have to be careful about taking certain medications, such as kutapressin, cold tablets, and nasal decongestants. Your physician can inform you of all the precautions you need to be concerned about when taking an MAO inhibitor. You should ask your doctor about Procardia, a drug that can quickly bring relief during a hypertensive crisis.

Shawn and I tried Nardil. Shawn didn't experience any improvement, but I did. This was one of the very few treatments that had any impact on my condition. Unfortunately, the benefit of increased energy was outweighed by the side effects. I felt as if I were in a manic state, unable to slow down, even when I felt sick. This continued until I was so completely worn out I had to discontinue treatment. I also experienced dizziness and vertigo.

## SEROTONIN RE-UPTAKE INHIBITORS (SRIs)

A third class of antidepressants, called serotonin re-uptake inhibitors (SRIs) are the newest class of antidepressant medications. They are popular now because they usually cause fewer side effects than the older antidepressants. Prozac and Zoloft are two of the more well known SRIs. I responded very well to Prozac. However, since I was also struggling with depression at that time, I am unable to determine if it treated my depression, my CFS, or both. Shawn saw an improvement in her sleep pattern on Zoloft. She went from sleeping fourteen hours a night to only nine or ten.

# EXERCISE

There is nothing more vital, yet seemingly unachievable, to the CFS patient than exercise. Ask any doctor and he or she will tell you that we need exercise because of the debilitating effects of long-term deconditioning. Even world-class athletes who are bedridden for a week can require months of reconditioning before they are back to full speed.

Prolonged bed rest is disastrous for the human body. It can

cause a loss of calcium and potassium, blood pooling, diminished lung capacity, mood disorders, fatigue, loss of muscle strength, hormone deficiencies, and a myriad of other problems. Only exercise can counteract the degenerative effect of a sedentary lifestyle, yet this presents a quandary for many of us. We are disabled and therefore unable to exercise, yet a lack of exercise contributes to our disability.

To address this, I went to a physical therapist to see if there was some sort of exercise regimen for people with my condition. Since I wasn't missing a limb or in a wheelchair and I looked normal, she started me on a program that was beyond my ability. In fact, she couldn't even do some of the exercises very well, which left me wondering, What good will these exercises do me when a healthy person can't even do them? But then it hit me: I have to do more than a healthy person just to break even. It is like a blind person needing a more acute sense of hearing to function better in this world.

The key was to develop a program and a pace that would build me up rather than wear me out. My inclination in anything athletic is to push myself as hard as I can as fast as I can, but this is a recipe for disaster with CFS. I must confess that I felt terribly wimpy riding on an exercise bike with no tension for a grand total of sixty seconds a day. But attempting anything more invariably left me relapsed and fatigued. I had to discover the line that divided benefit from detriment, a line that fluctuated depending on the kind of day I was having, as well as how much my conditioning had improved. This line is subjective for any of us, but it must be respected, for to cross it invites certain relapse. For anyone, especially the chronically ill, exercise is as vital to health as food and water. Make exercise a priority and set realistic goals, working with a doctor or a therapist. Learn to value quality over quantity, for anything gained is always better than grandiose planning that is not realized. And above all, try to be consistent.

# TREATING NEURALLY MEDIATED HYPOTENSION

As described in Chapter 4, "Understanding Your Illness," it is believed that some patients with CFS suffer from a condition called neurally medicated hypotension. Since this condition causes such similar symptoms to CFS—light-headedness, dizziness, weakness, and fatigue—it is very easy for doctors to miss this diagnosis. In short, this is a condition in which there is a dysfunction in your body's ability to control blood-pressure responses. For example, when a person without this condition arises from bed in the morning, the increased demand for blood due to the effects of gravity and movement is responded to with an increase in the heart rate and blood pressure so that blood is adequately distributed to the whole body. In people with hypotension, however, the opposite occurs. Just when you need the increased blood supply most, there is a decrease in blood pressure and heart rate, leaving your blood pooled where you need it least—in your legs. The lack of blood flow to the brain is what leaves you feeling dizzy and light-headed.

There are tests that doctors can perform to determine if you suffer from this condition. For example, they measure your circulatory response to varying conditions on a special table that tilts in different positions. But it is the treatment of this condition that I would like to focus on.

To counter the effects of hypotension you have to make it easier on your circulatory system to respond to increased workloads by increasing the volume of blood in your body. This ensures that the heart always has an ample supply of blood whenever it needs it. To achieve this, patients are typically given a medicine, such as Florinef, which helps the kidneys retain salt, which in turn helps the body retain fluids. Patients are also encouraged to drink more water and eat salty foods, which act as a natural fluid retainer.

Shawn was diagnosed four years ago with a related condition by the Mayo Clinic. It is unknown why she developed this condition, although one doctor thought it might have been due, in part, to the many years of deconditioning from CFS. She has responded incredibly well to the treatment regimen they proposed, and she no longer feels the racing heartbeat or sudden drops in blood pressure she had been experiencing. This has improved her level of functioning considerably. She has been able to avoid taking any medications simply by increasing her intake of salt, although to do so she needs to take so many salt tablets that occasionally her stomach becomes upset, leading to nausea and vomiting. That much salt is way beyond my ability to tolerate. Therefore, I am taking Florinef to treat my neurally mediated hypotension, and tolerating it quite well.

Shawn was also encouraged to exercise in order to improve circulation. She was told to wear support stockings to prevent the natural tendency of blood to pool in the legs due to the force of gravity.

The chief benefit I have felt from treating NMH is that I no longer feel as weak. It seems to give me more endurance and strength. This allows me to exercise more, as well as to tolerate activities that would have been impossible to undertake without my medicine.

## TREATMENT OF SLEEP DISORDERS

It is sadly ironic that for sufferers of a syndrome noted for excessive fatigue and sleep, improving our sleep should be one of our highest goals. Most CFS patients do have some type of sleep disturbance—they have trouble sleeping or they awaken completely unrefreshed. The use of low-dose tricyclic antidepressants has benefited many patients in this area.

I am convinced that some people with CFS not only have sleep disturbance, but also have a diagnosable type of sleep disorder. In fact, it may be the culprit behind some of their symptoms. We may not be able to recognize if we have developed a sleep disorder because, over the course of our illness, the symptoms of any sleep disorder can be so similar to CFS that they merge into one indistinguishable knot. It is important to recognize this, and to be tested, because oftentimes sleep disorders are treatable. There remains a need for future research to determine whether there is any correlation between CFS and sleep disorders, but since I am aware of many CFS patients who have developed sleep disorders, I proceed on the assumption that there may be.

Several years after we first became ill, we both developed noticeable sleep disorders. We were evaluated at sleep disorder centers, both locally and at the National Institutes of Health, and they found verifiable sleep disorders in both of us. We were connected to dozens of wires and electrodes to monitor our brain and muscle activities during the night. We then slept connected to a computer, which recorded our results. It was based on these results that a diagnosis was made.

During one of Shawn's nights at the center, she slept a total of 26 minutes with a sleep efficiency of 6 percent, which indicates severely disturbed sleep. During that 26 minutes, she had 18 uncontrolled leg movements for which she was diagnosed as having nocturnal myoclonus—uncontrollable leg twitches that cause disruptions in the natural rhythm of sleep, at all hours of the night. The next night, after being sleep deprived, Shawn slept 15 hours straight until they had to wake her. She felt she had slept soundly and was not aware that her legs were twitching the whole night. Being monitored allowed the doctors to observe that she was having leg movements, sometimes as often as every 20 seconds, throughout the night. This could easily explain part of the reason why she is unable to achieve restorative sleep.

I was found to have two problems that were different from Shawn's. First, I experienced "night terrors," a condition in which I wake up during the middle of the night totally disoriented and unaware of my surroundings. It is similar to sleep-walking in that I appear to be awake and can carry on a conversation with Shawn, not even realizing I am asleep. This disorder is usually seen in children. Second, I had difficulty with the rate of time it took me to go through the different stages of sleep, especially stage four, the deepest and most restorative period. I entered the different stages of sleep much too quickly, not spending enough time in each stage. Both of these contributed to a very poor night's sleep.

Something neither Shawn nor I have experienced, but which is another fairly common sleep disorder, is sleep apnea. People with this condition usually are not aware that they stop breathing momentarily throughout the night. Each time this happens, their sleep is disrupted. Many people who have sleep apnea also snore.

Many people don't realize they can have a sleep disorder and not be aware of it. If you momentarily stop breathing or experience leg twitches while you are asleep, your spouse may be the only one who will notice. Therefore, I recommend going to a sleep disorder center if there is the slightest hint of any type of problem.

Treatment for sleep disorders usually entails a multifaceted approach. Medicines such as Klonopin are given to minimize leg twitching or night terrors, and Sinequan aids in restorative sleep. Emphasis is also placed on changing behaviors that affect sleep. For instance, I have found that following a routine every night before I go to bed aids my sleep. It's as if our internal clock functions better on a schedule. I typically spend about forty-five minutes at night by myself, unwinding from the day, letting all my cares and worries slip away. I take a hot bath, which helps soothe my feelings and relax my nerves. I listen to soothing music and spend some time praying. I also try to go to sleep at roughly the same time each night to get my body used to falling asleep. I try to avoid stimulants such as caffeine before going to bed.

Another thing I have found quite helpful is taking a nap. Ever since I was a little kid I hated naps, but recently I have found them to be quite beneficial. In fact, I would rather sleep ten hours at night and take a two-hour nap during the day than sleep twelve hours at night. I seem to feel better this way. However, we are all different and some people do not sleep as well at night if they nap during the day.

We have also found a noisemaker to be very beneficial. My father-in-law bought us a special one from a catalog, but basically it's nothing more than a little fan in an enclosed chamber that makes a constant whirring sound during the night. It blocks out any other noises that might disturb our sleep.

## VITAMINS

The therapeutic value of vitamins in treating illness has been hotly debated for years. I have heard soul-stirring testimonies chronicling the miraculous recuperative power of vitamins. And, in fact, I do believe some of these accounts. Linus Pauling, a noted scientist and Nobel laureate, swore to their efficacy, and Norman Cousins, a well-respected author, believes that they literally saved his life.

The basic need for vitamins is not in dispute. Everyone needs them in order to live. By definition, vitamins are essential nutrients that must be obtained externally; the body is not able to manufacture them on its own. What is disputed is whether or not enough of these essential vitamins can be obtained solely from the food we eat. Do we need to supplement our diet with vitamin pills?

This question, like most questions concerning the fundamental mysteries of life, is beyond my ability to answer. (I can't even figure out why I always get full eating broccoli but never eating ice cream!) It is unfortunate that doctors, whose opinions we value most, are often undereducated in the field of nutrition.

It is equally unfortunate that the people who have the most training in nutrition may also have the greatest financial interest in pushing vitamins.

I believe in taking vitamin supplements for a number of reasons. Not a month goes by when you don't hear of some new scientific study touting the beneficial effects of vitamins. Just recently, folic acid has been proven to be helpful in preventing birth defects, and I read that pizza can help prevent cancer. Actually, it is some vitamin or nutrient in tomato sauce, but "Pizza Cures" makes for a much catchier headline.

I look at it this way: If I use the analogy of my body being a house, then CFS is a raging fire consuming that house. Some people scoff at vitamin therapy because they want proof that vitamins, like firemen, can put out the blaze. Unfortunately, their effect is much more subtle than that. To continue the analogy, I look at vitamins as enhancing the structure of my house. It means I have brick walls instead of wooden ones, and a foundation that is strong instead of weak. Therefore, the house is not as susceptible to the damage of flames. It doesn't put out the fire, but it sure makes being on fire less damaging.

It also stands to reason that what is sufficient for a healthy person may not be sufficient for someone who is sick. We may need more vitamins the same way a distance runner needs more fluid than the average person. Typically, most doctors only prescribe vitamins when a deficiency can be documented. But while we may not be demonstratively deficient, we may be functionally deficient. In other words, though our tests might all come back in the normal range, maybe that range is not adequate for us.

Recently, vitamin deficiencies have been linked to a whole slew of ailments. Lack of B-12 can cause nervous-system disorders ranging from muscle weakness to mental illness. Blood samples taken from people who had lung cancer were found to have significantly lower blood levels of vitamin E. I realize that this does not mean that consuming higher levels of vitamins can prevent lung cancer or cure mental illness. There may be a dysfunction in the utilization of vitamins, in which case any vitamins you take would simply be eliminated from the body without being absorbed.

For me, though, there is enough evidence that vitamins can be beneficial to encourage me to take them. I am, however, still leery of thinking of vitamins as miracle cures rather than supplements to better my health. I think this wariness came from the time my mother and I went to a special clinic for vitamin therapy. We went through the full regimen of expensive blood tests to determine which specific vitamins we were deficient in, as well as which ones might improve our health. We spent well over $600 and were taking up to 40 vitamins a day. I stopped taking the vitamins after several months because they had no noticeable effect and were very expensive.

Now, I take the more general, inexpensive vitamins. I no longer rush out to take the newest fad vitamin, but I do take the basic ones because I feel it contributes to my sense of well-being.

The hardest part of taking vitamins is figuring out which ones to take and how many. You should talk to your doctor before taking large doses of vitamins. Some, such as the A vitamins, can be toxic to your system when taken in large quantities. You should try to take a sufficient quantity to be beneficial, without taking so much you are wasting your time and money. We were fortunate to find a molecular biologist who has spent decades helping people improve their health with vitamin therapy, and he does it without the need for special, expensive tests. I take all the basics such as vitamins A, B, and E, but there are also some special vitamins and supplements that he recommends:

1. L-lysine is purported to be effective in fighting viral infections.
2. Vitamin C is heralded as a cure for everything from colds to cancer. Norman Cousins has written a book documenting his miraculous cure from cancer by using

megadoses of this vitamin. Shawn and I tried taking up to 25 grams a day of vitamin C, but now I am content to take much less. There are patients, however, who do claim some benefit from the more powerful intravenous form of vitamin C.

3. Riboflavin has been shown to be useful in treating migraines, from which I suffer.

4. B-12 has been reported to minimize fatigue in some CFS patients. Some people take it in oral form, but Shawn and I take B-12 injections. You need to take a multivitamin with B-12 to avoid vitamin imbalances.

5. Coenzyme Q10 acts like a catalyst for energy production in the cells. It is a naturally occurring nutrient that is administered to help with fatigue and muscle weakness. It is also believed to bolster the immune system.

6. Pycnogenol acts like a detoxifier, removing pollutants we encounter during our everyday lives. It also is a powerful antioxidant, which means it reduces the damaging effects of free radicals. These are renegade molecules, abnormal in chemical configuration, that are not supposed to be in your body.

7. Magnesium and malic acid are believed to be useful in improving cellular metabolism. They increase the utilization of substances necessary for energy production and are believed to be effective in reducing fatigue and muscle aches.

8. Melatonin, secreted by a gland in our body, is useful in aiding sleep. It has also been found to strengthen the immune system.

9. Germanium is believed to be able to improve utilization of oxygen in the tissues. It is also believed to induce the production of interferon, a product of the immune system that is necessary for fighting infection.

10. Primrose oil, an essential fatty acid necessary for healthy cell functioning, has been researched extensively in

Europe for this condition, with many positive results. It is believed to enhance the immune system and reduce fatigue and pain.

11. Beta carotene is believed to be able to increase natural killer cell activity, a possible problem in CFS patients.

12. L-Carnitine, available either by prescription or over the counter, is derived from lysine, an essential amino acid. It facilitates the transport of fatty acids to the mitochondria, which are then utilized for energy production.

## GAMMA GLOBULIN

There have not been double-blind placebo-controlled studies conducted to determine the efficacy of gamma globulin in treating CFS. While clinical trials have revealed conflicting findings, some people not only claim to feel better while they are on this treatment, but have regained their health as well.

As therapies go, gamma globulin has very few side effects and is not toxic to the body. However, the long-term use of very high doses of any medicine should never be undertaken lightly.

Gamma globulin is a concentration of some of the antibodies found in blood. The name gamma globulin is another name for immunoglobulin, or antibodies. It is a blood product that is prepared by distilling, concentrating, and purifying the antibodies from the blood plasma (a part of the blood that doesn't contain any cells) of many different donors. It has a very high concentration of immunoglobulin G, known also as IgG, and lesser concentrations of other antibodies.

Specific antibodies are necessary to destroy specific viruses. If the body is deficient in some of these antibodies, it may be unable to control certain infections. Gamma globulin is given in the hope that it will replace whatever antibodies may be deficient. In this way, antibodies are transferred from one person to another, passing immunity from one to another.

This treatment may be especially beneficial for CFS patients who exhibit a deficiency in neutralizing antibodies of one or more of the subclasses of IgG antibodies. IgG can be divided into four subclasses, and some patients with CFS exhibit a deficiency in one of these four subclasses. Doctors are still not certain how much significance to place on subclass deficiency since the overall IgG levels in CFS patients are usually normal. But since gamma globulin does contain neutralizing antibodies as well as all four subclasses of IgG, in theory this treatment could help.

Gamma globulin can be given either intravenously (IV) or by injection. Intravenous treatment is the preferred method because it delivers a greater amount of the medicine than does injection. If you receive this medicine intravenously, be prepared to spend quite a few hours at the hospital. There is a lot of medicine to be given, and it should be administered slowly to avoid any side effects. With any infusion, there is always a possibility of experiencing an adverse reaction. The rapid infusion of gamma globulin may induce an inflammatory or allergic response, such as fever, headache, chills, and nausea. Even though serious reactions are unusual, patients should be carefully monitored during their treatments.

The dosage of gamma globulin is weight dependent; the more you weigh, the greater the amount of medicine you will receive. I started at a low dosage and continued to increase it to the maximum allowed within safe limits. Your physician can inform you of all the specifics.

One drawback of gamma globulin is that it is very expensive. When my wife and I were receiving the highest doses, the annual cost of the treatment was over $25,000 for each of us. Fortunately, we were both covered by insurance, so we did not have to worry about the bills. But if you are not as fortunate, you should discuss your financial limitations with the hospital. Many hospitals make special arrangements for people who are in financial need. They frequently operate on a sliding scale; you pay according to what you can afford. So don't assume this treatment isn't available to you because of its cost.

Gamma globulin may be very slow in taking effect. Some patients see an improvement in two or three months, but others not for over a year. This was one of the very first treatments Shawn and I received, and it was during the worst time of our illness. We tried this treatment for approximately one and a half years, but to no avail. I do know people with CFS, however, who claim to have been helped dramatically by this treatment.

Because gamma globulin is derived from a blood product, I think it is important that I discuss a concern on everybody's mind these days: AIDS. With the raging paranoia surrounding this deadly disease, people are understandably reticent to use anything that is derived from a blood product. I know I was. Of course, no doctor can give you a blanket guarantee, but mine assured me that the chance of contracting AIDS from gamma globulin is virtually nonexistent.

Almost all of the AIDS cases that have resulted from contaminated blood have been from transfusions of whole blood. Gamma globulin is considered safe not only because blood donors are now well screened for AIDS, but also because it uses just a small fraction of the blood, which is processed through many stages of filtering, distillation, and purification. There is very little chance that the virus associated with AIDS could still remain.

Gamma globulin has been used for decades in treating immunodeficient patients, people who display an inadequate amount of certain immune cells. As of this writing, my doctor knows of no reported AIDS cases being linked to the use of this treatment. But this is still a question that only you can resolve. You, and you alone, have to weigh even the remote possibility of risk against the possible benefits.

# TRANSFER FACTOR

Transfer factor is a treatment that neither my wife nor I have tried, but we have heard enough anecdotal evidence that we would consider trying it in the future. There has been some research conducted on the use of transfer factor for chronic fatigue syndrome, but there have not been any controlled, double-blind studies. Therefore, while some research findings indicate potential benefit from using this medicine, others do not, and this medicine has never risen to the forefront of treatments for CFS. We know of a physician with CFS who has found it extremely beneficial.

Transfer factor is considered safe as far as side effects are concerned. It has been used for quite a few years, and most of its possible side effects are known. It is a blood product, however, and therefore there is a concern about AIDS. Transfer factor is not considered as safe as gamma globulin because it does not go through as many stages of purification as gamma globulin does, so even greater caution is necessary. Donors should be well screened for both hepatitis and AIDS.

Transfer factor is derived from the immune system, but it is not antibodies. It is believed to be a lymphokine product that is secreted by white blood cells to help fight infection. If CFS is caused by an inability to fight infection, this treatment may enable the immune system to learn this ability. It is hoped that this medicine "transfers" the ability to fight CFS from someone who has successfully recovered from this syndrome to someone who has not.

If patients with CFS are missing some vital genetic or chemical piece of information, preventing the immune system from recognizing or controlling this illness, maybe that missing piece can be supplied by the transfer factor. In a sense, transfer factor teaches the immune system what to do. It causes the unsensitized white blood cells to become sensitized and better qualified to deal with infections. In other words, it transforms general lymphocytes into lethal ones.

This drug is injected intramuscularly, and it may require several injections before it takes effect. Once it does, the injections should not need to be continued as often. Once the immune system has been sensitized, it can recall this information. However, infrequent follow-up treatments will probably be necessary to maintain the improvement.

## DIET

This is one area I am quite familiar with. There is hardly a diet claiming even the slightest therapeutic value that I haven't tried. The purpose of these diets is not weight loss, although this is usually claimed as an extra benefit. Rather, these diets are supposed to enable the body to function in a healthier manner.

Some of these diets claim to bolster the immune system. They hold that there are certain food groups, such as wheat, soy, and dairy products, that can cause allergic reactions. The immune system, which is the primary system involved in any type of allergic reaction, is weakened by these foods. You feel ill because your body is mistaking these foods for foreign invaders, attacking them as it would a virus. These strict diets eliminate the suspect foods, and also claim that other foods can actually bolster the immune system.

Another diet that is popular is the yeast-free diet. Yeast, like bacteria, is normally found in the body and, in small quantities, poses no threat. However, if your immunity is low and yeast multiplies unchecked, a yeast infection could be triggered, making you ill. You put out the "fire" by eliminating the fuel. Anything containing yeast is completely restricted. I was amazed to learn how prevalent yeast is. It is found not only in bread, but in pasteurized milk, many vitamins, cheese, canned goods, alcohol, enriched pasta, and a host of other food products. Since yeast feeds on sugar, any foods containing sugar must also be eliminated.

Even though we did not improve through these diets, we felt as if it was an important step in ruling out yeast infections and food allergies. If you do unknowingly suffer from food allergies or yeast infections, these diets may, in fact, be very beneficial.

There are many other health-conscious diets, and while we have not been cured on any of them, our bodies do seem to function better when we are eating better. After all, common sense tells us that it has to be healthier to eat cauliflower than candy. We try to combine the nutritionally sound information from all of these diets. We still love our ice cream, but we eat many more fruits and vegetables than we used to. Although diets may not cure CFS, proper nutrition is essential to enable the body to function, much less heal itself. Our only source of energy comes from the food we eat, therefore, it is essential that we maintain proper nutrition. You may feel a step stronger just from changing your diet and eating more nutritious meals.

## CLINICAL ECOLOGY

Clinical ecologists believe that the environment can literally make a person ill. The chemicals in tap water may be polluting your body. The food you eat may be causing allergic reactions and suppressing your immune system. Even the air you breathe may be filled with harmful chemicals. Nothing is free from suspicion. They believe that environmental stresses overload the immune system and increase susceptibility to disease.

Shawn and I went to a clinical ecologist in New York City. We underwent extensive testing to determine what we were allergic to, as well as what toxic chemicals might be making us ill. Aside from suggesting changes of diet and environment, this clinical ecologist gave us nystatin, an antifungal drug, to control yeast infections. He also claimed to have had a lot of success using injections of flu vaccine, which he said encouraged the production of antibodies that relieve certain symptoms associated with CFS.

I really do believe that the environment can make a person ill, and that taking steps to eliminate toxins, allergens, and poisons from one's environment can only be beneficial. In addition, we have heard from CFS patients who have been helped by clinical ecologists. However, Shawn and I spent a lot of money without receiving any noticeable benefit.

## CHIROPRACTIC

For financial reasons, I have not been under chiropractic care for many years. If I could afford it, however, I would still be going. It's not that chiropractic care can cure my CFS, but rather that I simply felt better while under it. Chiropractors do not seek to cure any specific illness, or even merely to relieve backaches, as is commonly believed. Their stated purpose is to allow the body to function at its best.

Nerves connect every organ of the body to enable them to function together as one unit. The theory behind chiropractic care is that when those nerves are pinched, they become like a hose with a kink, unable to let the water of life flow through. Nerves become pinched when the bones of the spine become twisted or misaligned. This is referred to as a vertebral subluxation. Chiropractors manipulate these bones back into their normal positions, thereby removing the pressure on the nerves. When the nerves are free from any interference, every part of the body will be able to function in a healthier manner.

Whatever your feelings on the philosophy of chiropractic care, Shawn and I noticed some significant changes when we were receiving it. Though they are unrelated to CFS, many of the aches and pains we used to put up with disappeared.

## ACUPUNCTURE

Acupuncture is similar to chiropractic in its belief in the body's innate intelligence to heal itself. Rather than manipulating the spine, however, acupuncturists insert very fine needles into strategic areas of the body. Disease results from a blockage of these points, and health will only be restored when the balance of the body is restored.

There is some scientific evidence to support the claims of acupuncture. For example, the human body is able to produce natural painkillers and hormones that are vital to a state of health. It is believed that the insertion of the needles stimulates the release of these chemicals, thereby making you feel better.

Shawn and I underwent acupuncture treatments for months, but did not see any change in the symptoms of CFS.

## THE POWER OF POSITIVE THINKING

There are many headings I could have given this section, but whatever the name, many people find that their attitudes and beliefs affect their illness. The reason I am including this in the chapter on treatments is that it is believed people have the ability to influence and alter their state of health, to some degree, either positively or negatively. For example, it is known that daily stress can suppress the immune system, thereby making the body vulnerable to infection. Therefore, it is believed you can improve your health by eliminating stress, having a positive mental attitude, and visualizing that you are getting well. I want to make it clear that I am not referring to psychic healing using New Age techniques, but rather an alteration in the way we think and feel about ourselves in order to promote better health.

There are scores of books dealing with this subject, so I am not going to go into great detail. For example, some books believe that laughter is good medicine. It is known that laughter causes the release of chemicals from the brain that help reduce inflammation and ease pain. Norman Cousins partially attributes his remarkable recovery from cancer to this theory. He put it into practice by watching funny movies, such as old Marx Brothers films. Science has learned from the placebo effect that the mind is a powerful force. Therefore, if you create positive mental and emotional images, you may be able to influence your illness.

To be honest, I am not sure how I feel about these types of therapies. Shawn and I tried many different techniques to visualize ourselves well, but we invariably experienced feelings of frustration and failure when we weren't cured. Because these techniques tended to put all the responsibility for our illness onto us, they resulted in emotional turmoil, the opposite of what the techniques were supposed to accomplish.

I know that what we believe does in some way affect how we feel. I am just not ready to make the leap in logic that we therefore have total control over our bodies by what we think and feel. I no longer look upon positive thinking as a potential cure for CFS, but, as with exercise and good nutrition, I see it as an additional way to improve my health. At the very least, a positive rather than a negative attitude is very important in coping with this illness.

## HOMEOPATHY

Homeopathy is an alternative healing science that uses medicines to help the body heal itself. Some of the medicines used are herbs, roots, oils, minerals, and vitamins, but the most controversial is the use of microdoses of compounds that are typically associated with the cause of a disease, not the cure of it. Homeopathy literally means "same suffering," for it is believed that what causes a problem is what cures a problem. For example, if you suffer from allergies to bee stings, you are given minute doses of bee venom.

In fact, these doses are so small that not a single molecule of whatever particular treatment you are trying is even detectable. The theory is that the water holding each particular treatment is able to memorize the imprint of a substance and transfer that memory to the patient. I do not know if homeopathy is able to relieve any of the symptoms of CFS, but I do know that a year of treatment did not result in any improvement for Shawn or me. There remain, however, many people with CFS who claim to benefit from homeopathy.

## ACYCLOVIR (ZOVIRAX)

Acyclovir is one of the new generation of antiviral drugs available today. The effectiveness of this drug for CFS was tested by the National Institutes of Health and was found to be no more effective than a placebo, but I mention it because I learned a lot being a part of this study. Both Shawn and I have received IV and oral acyclovir. I received it as part of a double-blind study conducted by the NIH. A double-blind study is a scientifically controlled study to ascertain objectively the efficacy of a drug. It is called double-blind because neither the patient nor the doctor knows when the drug is being given and when the placebo is given (a placebo is nothing more than a sugar pill and has no medicinal value). Administering drugs and placebos at different times or to different patients allows doctors to discover whether patients are feeling better simply because they believe the medicine can cure them, or because of the effect of the medicine itself. If the majority of patients feel better on the medicine and not the placebo, doctors can be sure that the medicine does, in fact, work. The placebo effect is a very interesting phenomenon; the mind is tricked into healing the body. Some people in my study experienced the placebo effect. At first I was terribly disappointed to learn that people with my illness tricked themselves into feeling better. I couldn't help thinking that if patients got well on nothing more than a sugar pill, fuel would be added to the fire of disbelief. It is bad enough that so many people think CFS is all in our minds without giving them the proof to back up their claim. Then I realized that I was looking at this phenomenon the wrong way. Instead of regarding the placebo effect as a threat to the authenticity of my illness, I began to look at it as a wonderful testament to the power of hope and belief. The brain is a marvelous organ, an unexplored treasure trove of healing riches. The innate intelligence to make us feel better is within our own bodies. We actually have the power to affect our own health. I am not suggesting that, like Peter Pan, we merely need to think happy thoughts. But the placebo effect does prove that we can have a positive impact on the way we feel. I received intravenous acyclovir in the hospital, three times a day for seven days. The intravenous form of the drug is very powerful and gives this medicine the best possible chance of working. Immediately following this intravenous treatment, I took the less potent oral form of the drug for four weeks. Unfortunately, I did not feel better on either trial. In fact, the only way I could tell the difference between the drug and the placebo was that I felt worse on the drug. There are patients, however, who do claim to feel better on this medicine. At present, Dr. Straus of the NIH cannot recommend acyclovir because he did not find it effective in placebo-controlled trials.

## AGGRESSIVE REST THERAPY (ART)

My father-in-law, John Barlass, deserves all the credit for the development of this ingenious therapy. He could see that, though it was painstakingly slow, we did seem to improve gradually as we rested. He observed that it was only after we were confined to the house, literally unable to do anything for a year and a half, that we started regaining our strength.

He realized that none of the treatments or medications we tried had been able to make us well. He also noticed that activity always made us worse—that only by resting were we able to lessen the severity of our symptoms. From this he theorized that since rest lessened the severity of our symptoms, it might also be the key to actually making us well. We were so busy chasing after experimental therapies that we were never able to give our bodies the rest they desperately cried out for. He also believed that our bodies have an innate ability to heal themselves, and should be given every chance to do so.

From this humble beginning arose a unique treatment for CFS: aggressive rest therapy (ART). We were not to do anything other than rest. The concept of ART is not just to rest when you feel horribly ill or even merely to eliminate "pushing"; this is a program of aggressive rest. Even when you feel you have a little energy, you should rest. In fact, you should rest all the time. There were only two exceptions to this. One was to exercise in order to prevent deconditioning, and the other was to do enough to meet our emotional and psychological needs, such as visiting with a friend.

This is probably the most difficult thing you will ever do. It is not easy to rest aggressively, even for people with CFS who are completely exhausted. Whenever you get a little bit of energy, you want to use it before you lose it. With ART, however, you should not put that energy to use for anything but letting your body heal.

This means that you have to curtail all but the essential activities. You will need help with grocery shopping, errands, preparing meals, laundry, cleaning, and so on. For this you may need the help of family and friends, or you may even have to hire someone if you can afford to. You may want to contact the churches in your area; they may be able to suggest someone who can help you for a reasonable fee or even donate their services. I offer further suggestions in Chapter 7, "Coping with Your Illness."

In the beginning, it is difficult to rest aggressively because you worry about all the things you think you should be doing. You need to regard resting as you do medication. In order for medicine to be effective, you must take it faithfully. In the same manner, you must be faithful to your resting therapy. In order to do this, you have to disregard the unrealistic expectations imposed on you by others as well as by yourself. You are no longer able to do many, if not most, of the things you used to do. Though you may feel that you have no alternative but to continue pushing yourself beyond your limits, in fact, you do have choices. If you broke your ankles you would be forced to rest. You decide every day what you will spend your energy and strength on. It is amazing how your life changes once you realize how many choices you truly have.

At the end of three months (the minimum amount of time we give each new therapy) we evaluated the effectiveness of ART. I must admit that both Shawn and I did feel better. I am not going to say that by aggressively resting you will get well. You may, but I have no evidence either way. However, we discovered that our illness was much easier to cope with when we were resting. We found that our symptoms were not as severe and we were not as irritable, having more to give to our relationship.

The theory behind ART is that it allows you to rest, and that allows you to take some control over your illness. Resting is not giving in; it is taking an active and aggressive approach, and from your letters I think most of you agree. We received more feedback about ART than anything else I wrote about in the first edition of this book.

I honestly feel that this therapy was a lifesaver for me. I was beginning to feel like a frayed rope, ready to unravel and snap. Thanks to ART, I feel I have some semblance of a life again. Some people with CFS are not completely debilitated and find they can cope without such a restrictive lifestyle. While ART didn't cure us, it did help us change our lifestyle dramatically, changing the way we spend our energy. We also retreat back into "mini ART" whenever we relapse.

We have seen how much we hurt ourselves with too much activity, and ART has helped us to learn to limit ourselves much more. This has helped to prevent the severe relapses and made coping more manageable. Therefore, even if you are only able to implement ART in small ways, you will find it very beneficial.

In addition to the treatments I have described, some people try to alleviate their symptoms with other medications, such as antianxiety drugs, sedatives, muscle relaxants, aspirin, nonnarcotic analgesics, antihistamines, antipyretics for fever, and others. There are also many health products that people try, including barley green, royal jelly, primrose oil, germanium, coenzyme Q10, and others. This list is not exhaustive by any means. Only you and your doctor can evaluate the effectiveness of these treatments in relieving some of your symptoms. Do not try any treatment without consulting your doctor first.

With any treatment, it is difficult to be sure whether you are taking the right dosage for a long enough period of time. Shawn and I usually build up to the safest maximum dosage of anything we try and give a treatment a minimum of three months in which to be effective. Up until a few years ago, physicians did not have uniform diagnostic criteria by which to compare their patients with the patients of other researchers. As a result, anecdotal accounts of miraculous cures have often spread, only to have it turn out that the people who got well never even had CFS. By the same token, therapies dismissed in the past as useless for CFS need to be reevaluated because they might have been ineffective for precisely the same reason.

I know I have given you a lot to think about. If you have just recently been diagnosed as having CFS, the choice of treatments may seem overwhelming. Don't rush into any treatment.

Discuss all your options with your doctor, weighing the risks against the benefits. Some people with CFS are able to manage their illness without the use of medication. If you cannot, carefully choose the treatment that you are most comfortable with. Do not be discouraged if one treatment does not seem to help, because maybe another one will.

# Depression and Chronic Fatigue Syndrome

*As a CFS sufferer, I have discovered that the symptom of depression has a physical as well as a psychological dimension. CFS has manifested itself physically by debilitating me. It has depressed me in the very literal sense that it has severely limited my strength and activity. In addition to this, the constant pain and frustration of a chronic illness like CFS can also have a profound impact on a sufferer, resulting in emotional depression.*

This is a very intimidating chapter for me to write. The mere possibility that depression plays any role in chronic fatigue syndrome represents such a painful and emotional issue for sufferers of this illness that I am more than a little reluctant to share my experiences on the matter. I want to be completely open and honest, yet I don't want to stigmatize further people whose illness is discounted as merely psychosomatic. If my experience is typical, however, I must confess that depression may play some role in CFS. And that experience has convinced me that I did not fully understand this subject when I wrote about it many years ago. It's not that what I wrote wasn't true, rather I had no concept of just how true these words were. In the previous edition of this book, depression was listed as merely one of many symptoms, barely comprising one page. I realize now that such a meager treatment of so pervading a symptom was, at best, wholly inadequate.

For the last few years I have been struggling with clinically diagnosed, full-blown depression, and it has given me a new perspective on its relationship to CFS. On one hand, depression is not the same as chronic fatigue syndrome. And most anyone who has had both can tell the difference. On the other hand, I truly believe that depression can play a role in CFS, albeit a secondary one. Conflicting assertions? On the surface it may seem so, but upon closer examination they are complementary, not contradictory. In hindsight, I can now see how a low level of depression may have made many of my CFS symptoms worse. It was not the cause of my symptoms, but it did tend to exacerbate and amplify them. In the same way that pneumonia is not the cause of AIDS, but an opportunistic infection that plagues AIDS patients, depression, while not the cause of CFS, is an opportunistic defection that can plague CFS patients.

How can one tell the difference? Simply put, CFS often makes me feel as if I don't have the strength to live, while depression makes me feel as if I don't have the strength to want to live. This distinction is not subtle. CFS robs you of your strength and poisons your body; depression robs you of your will and poisons your spirit. In addition, people with depression usually have very little self-awareness, while CFS patients tend to be so in tune with their bodies that they sometimes appear fanatical. People with depression often don't seek medical help on their own, yet CFS patients are relentless in their pursuit of anything that will improve their health.

Recent research seems to confirm that there is a distinction between CFS and depression as well. Subtle immunologic and hormonal imbalances have been discovered in CFS patients that are not usually found in people with classic melancholic depression. The NIH did research on levels of cortisol (a naturally occurring hormone) in CFS patients and found them to be low, the opposite of what is seen in people with clinical depression. The typical CFS patient does not meet the criteria for diagnosis of depression and does not recover from treatment with antidepressants. In addition, physical findings such as tender lymph nodes and recurrent sore throats are not typically observed in patients with clinical depression.

There are physicians who claim that clinical depression, left untreated, can result in CFS. While this may or may not be true, I think the reverse is just as likely to occur. The emotional toll inflicted by CFS, left untreated, can lead to a major depression. I think that CFS-linked depression can be a combination of emotional distress (reactive depression) and chemical imbalances (endogenous depression). Reactive depression results from our intellectual and emotional inability to cope with stress. For example, how we manage long-term illness often determines the level of reactive depression we have to deal with. Endogenous depression results from a physical defect in our biochemical and hormonal systems. In other words, this type of depression is a physical illness, no different from diabetes.

Since I have had mild and severe depression, I feel as if I am in a unique position to comment on the differences between the two. It was not that long ago that I had a bout with severe depression. In fact, it was only three or four years ago that my mild depression slipped its restraining bonds and overwhelmed me to the point where I could barely function, let alone recover from it. I went for well over a decade of my illness with little concern for this psychiatric nightmare, therefore when it hit I was wholly unprepared for its calamitous effect. It followed a particularly traumatic relapse, and it took me a year and a half to recover fully from its effects.

I had been feeling better than I had felt in over a decade. I was not well, but my improvement was so remarkable I felt like a new person. I was taking a medication called kutapressin, the only treatment that had ever made a significant difference in my health. I was eating and sleeping better, and trying vitamins and supplements that seemed to give me an energy boost. I was also able to go to a physical therapist who was helping me exercise, moderately but regularly. I vowed to myself that I would do whatever it took never to go back to the way I was feeling during the past ten years.

Unfortunately, circumstances dictated differently. I fell prey to numerous colds and flus, which interrupted my exercise regimen. I also began to develop a slight heart problem, later diagnosed as mitral valve prolapse, which seemed to increase my level of fatigue. My doctor moved away and, because of financial limitations, as well as an inability to find a doctor to prescribe it for me, I was unable to continue taking kutapressin. I went without it for months and my health plummeted. As my strength spiraled downward, so did my psychological well-being. I became so depressed I couldn't even recognize what bad shape I was in, and Shawn practically had to force me to go to the doctor for an antidepressant.

However, looking back, I can see that the seeds of my depression were sown long before I became severely depressed. It just took a major stress, like a relapse, to push me over the edge. I believe that any type of mild depression or psychological dysfunction is a potential trigger mechanism for full-blown, severe depression. Whether you suffer from CFS or multiple sclerosis, chronic illness can cause depression. And the impact of depression can either contribute to the cycle of chronic illness or cause a major, clinical depression.

The worst part is, many of the warning signs leading up to severe depression can closely mimic symptoms associated with chronic illnesses like CFS. Fatigue, sadness, inability to enjoy usual activities, troubled thinking, inability to work, withdrawal, sleep problems, headaches, memory problems, and feelings of hopelessness are hallmarks of both conditions. That is one reason there is so much contention and confusion concerning the role of depression in CFS. But more than our credibility is at stake here. Minor depression, left untreated, can potentially lead to devastatingly severe clinical depression. Just as importantly, mild depression is often treatable, and the sooner it is recognized, the easier it is to treat.

In my case, I found it impossible to spend years being ill and not struggle with depression. Anyone suffering from any illness, chronic or acute, experiences some degree of depression. It is as natural an emotional response as crying when we have lost a loved one. Therefore, at least in part, my clinical depression was simply the manifestation and culmination of untreated mild depression brought about by a chronic, debilitating illness.

That is not to say that there isn't also a physical component to my depression as well. In fact, I was treated with Prozac without counseling or therapy and I recovered quite nicely. The Prozac remedied my chemical imbalances enough for me to deal with and work through all the varied emotions brought on by my relapse. Contrary to popular belief, antidepressants are not happy pills that will make anybody's life better. They do not control people, acting as some kind of drug-induced straitjacket. They are only effective in people who have chemical imbalances, correcting them the same way insulin corrects diabetes. In severe depression, a combination of counseling and medication is the most effective treatment.

Many people aren't aware that certain medications can cause depression. Shawn had a severe bout of depression that was brought about by the long-term use of prednisone for her asthma. We were surprised to find that after she discontinued the prednisone the depression did not lift, but our doctor said that once the chemicals in the brain are affected, they often won't return to normal on their own. Treatment with Zoloft brought Shawn out of her depression.

Depression is not something that you should allow to go untreated. It is very dangerous when it is suppressed and allowed to grow. It prevents clear and rational thinking, causing bitterness, self-absorption, hopelessness, and emotional instability. This destroys any chance you have of coping with your illness. Any chronic illness that is stressful and painful requires a constant struggle for emotional acceptance and adaptation. I found that I needed an outlet for the constant, daily barrages of discouragement and frustration, and it has been a real blessing for me to have a counselor to share with. Friends and family are a good source of support in this area, but they can't always be there in the way you might need. Therefore, don't be embarrassed to seek professional help. I realize that there has always been a stigma attached to seeing a counselor, making us feel weak or inadequate. However, the amount of energy we waste is enormous when we try to deny our problems instead of treating them.

I try to cope with depression by implementing four basic axioms, and perhaps they could be of help to you:

1. I try to cut myself some slack. When I tend to get down on myself, feeling that I am somehow to blame, this just increases my feelings of depression. Depression is not caused by personal weakness, therefore it can't be resisted through personal strength.
2. I remind myself that mild depression waxes and wanes. When I feel particularly blue, I try to hold on until a day when my mind and my emotions are a bit clearer.
3. I am training myself to accentuate the positive. I do things that make me feel happier and avoid things that bring me down.
4. I seek help. Typically, this takes the form of finding comfort from family and friends, but it also may entail seeking professional help. Remember, too, that you cannot just snap out of a severe depression by trying; sometimes medication is required.

# Coping with Your Illness

*Though the illness is strong, I must be stronger.*

Coping with chronic fatigue syndrome is one of the greatest challenges I have ever faced. The very problems and emotions I struggled to master yesterday come rushing back today with undiminished intensity. I feel as if I am in a desperate fight in which defeat is ever looming yet victory is never assured. It is only by taking each day, one day at a time, that I am able to withstand this unrelenting affliction. Not a day goes by that I am not bombarded with a myriad of burdensome emotions. Coping with CFS is an ongoing struggle that is never easy, but I have learned some things that may help you through.

One of the most important things any of us can do is to understand what we are up against. Understanding gives us the wisdom to know our foe and defeat it. I am not referring to a medical perspective, or to how CFS affects us physically, but rather, how CFS affects us mentally, emotionally, and spiritually. Learning how your illness affects you and understanding your reactions to it will make it easier to cope with. In other words, it is not enough to say that CFS makes me feel lousy. I have to identify what specifically is making me feel lousy at this moment, for example not having children, and acknowledge my reaction and response to that feeling, for example sadness. By doing this we can remedy, and to some degree prevent, much of the damage CFS inflicts, thereby reclaiming some measure of control over our lives. CFS is a very demanding illness, but its demands can be met. I hope that this chapter will help you meet the challenge.

## COPING MENTALLY

It took me the longest time to realize that of all the considerable burdens imposed on me by CFS, the weight of my own expectations was of millstone proportions. It was then a short leap in logic to the realization that the way I think about this illness has, to some extent, an impact on the effect of the illness. For example, when I constantly lamented the fact that I never finished seminary, CFS was a powerful entity that robbed me of my chance to make a difference in this world. But when I began focusing on the letters I received from people who were ministered to by the first edition of this book, some even forgoing suicide, CFS no longer had the power to take away my purpose in this world. My purpose is different, but I choose to think of it as no less significant. There are three crucial areas that anyone with CFS needs to come to terms with: redefining your sense of self-worth, accepting your new limitations, and redefining your priorities.

### REDEFINING YOUR SENSE OF WORTH

Often, a poor self-image is at the root of the difficulties people experience when coping with CFS. A poor self-image can be just as debilitating as any physical symptom and can exacerbate negative emotions. It is not difficult to understand why CFS is powerful enough to damage even the healthiest self-image. This illness may prevent you from being free and independent. You are no longer able to dictate to your body; it dictates to you. Perhaps you used to base your sense of worth on your accomplishments at work and at play. Now any achievements, even minor ones, may seem few and far between.

If you have a severe case of CFS, you are no longer able to be who you once were. The more you wish your illness would go away, the harder it will be to cope with. You have to admit to yourself that you have a chronic illness and, until such time as you get well, you will not be who you once were. You must put the past to rest. Grieve over it as you would grieve the loss of a loved one, but then let it go. You need to accept and even respect who you are now. By letting go of the past, you can cope better with the present.

At least for now, you need to build a new self. I knew who the old me was, and I dream of who the healed me will be, but now I have to concentrate on defining the present me. I accomplish this by doing what gives me a sense of fulfillment and purpose now, including activities I barely considered undertaking when I was well, such as doing a simple puzzle or growing plants. Your life may have changed, but it is no less significant. You must constantly remind yourself that you are important, and you may have to change ingrained attitudes about what constitutes self-worth.

Many people define themselves by their employment. When that employment is taken away, so is their identity. You may feel that your life is somehow less worthwhile because you can no longer measure your worth by the fruits of your labors. But a person's worth should not be assessed by the amount of money he or she has earned. I would much rather be respected for my investment in relationships than for my financial success.

Focus on your inner worth. Who you are is more important than what you do. By enduring this illness, you are developing a depth of character that others may never attain. You may be surprised at the precious qualities that unfold within you: patience, perseverance, understanding, self-control, empathy, and faith. Enduring pain and suffering may not seem noble at the time, only difficult. But in the end there can be no greater tribute paid to a person than to say that, with courage and humility, he or she bore the hardships of suffering.

Certainly don't let another person ruin your self-esteem. It doesn't matter what anyone else thinks about you or your illness. All that matters is that you realize how strong and brave you truly are. People understand only what they want to understand. Don't waste your precious strength trying to defend your status as a valued member of society.

A sense of competence and accomplishment is also important in maintaining your self-worth. Don't dwell on what you can no longer do; instead choose to focus on what you can. Be realistic about your limitations and avoid setting goals that you can't reach. Undertake small, easily accomplished tasks. If you are not bedridden, you may even consider taking up a small hobby, something that is not too draining but is satisfying.

Another necessary component of self-worth is a sense of belonging. It is a blessing to have supportive family and friends who acknowledge your pain and suffering. Rely on them to help you through this painful time in your life. I know how difficult it is to receive; I much prefer giving. But I have learned to accept the help of others graciously because I would not be able to survive without it.

Even with a loving support system, though, CFS may make it difficult for you to feel you truly belong. Consider contacting one of the CFS organizations listed in Appendix D, to find others with this illness whom you can meet or talk to. It is comforting to be with people who know what you are going through. A good support group can help build self-esteem, dispel fear and anxiety, and provide information and encouragement. You may also want to consider professional counseling to help you build self-esteem. Some of you may be reticent about seeking professional help because it is difficult for you to be open and honest with a stranger. After a while, however, a counselor is no longer a stranger but may, in fact, seem like a good friend.

## ACCEPTING YOUR LIMITATIONS

One of the most important new concepts I had to appropriate was: My body is not the enemy; it is merely a victim. I had to learn to understand and respect its limitations without feeling as if I was surrendering. I had to make the distinction that struggling against the ravages of CFS is not the same as blindly ignoring my body's need for rest. Our body has an innate intelligence. It sends messages that must be heeded, not ignored.

If you are disabled by CFS, the benefits of accepting a lifestyle of limited activity may seem obvious. Unfortunately, it took Shawn and me years before we were willing to accept this new lifestyle. We tried to ignore the limitations imposed by our illness and we were left barely hanging by an emotional thread.

We now determine whether or not an activity is worthwhile by how much strength and energy it requires. If it requires more than its potential benefit, it is not worth doing. I hope you learn from our mistake and choose to accept your limitations before you no longer have the choice. It may help to think about your limitations not as a sign of weakness, but as a beneficent truce.

Of course changing your lifestyle will be difficult. We spend our entire lives under the shadow of preconceived expectations. When Shawn and I were first married, she wanted and expected to fill the role of a homemaker and she felt guilty because she needed so much help. When you're chronically ill, though, your preconceived roles become meaningless and your only expectation should be to rest as much as possible so you have the strength to cope with your illness. For a long time we tried to live up to our old expectations, and we lived under a constant cloud of failure and frustration. It is not easy to lower your standards on everything in your life, from how you dress to cleaning your home, or even what birthday presents you can afford to buy for those you love. You want to function as you used to, but you will constantly feel inadequate and powerless unless you truly redefine and accept your limitations. Wearing wrinkled clothes and having a home that is less than spotless is a small price to pay for any improvement in your health.


## REDEFINE YOUR PRIORITIES

Adapting to a lifestyle of limited activity requires thought and imagination, as well as the ability to define priorities. To define your priorities, scrutinize every activity and eliminate all but the essential. It wasn't until we started ART (aggressive rest therapy, discussed in Chapter 5, "Treatments") that we began to change our thinking from "But we have to . . ." to "Do we have to . . . ?" We examined every activity, realized how much of our precious strength was being stolen by unnecessary endeavors, and eliminated all but the most important.

At first we felt selfish for choosing only the activities that were important to us, but we knew it was a physical and emotional necessity. Now we have struck a balance by occasionally doing what others want, even if it is not in our best interest. All in all, though, we have cut down on our activities tremendously. This new lifestyle minimizes our physical pain and keeps us emotionally sane, which is just as important to our health as any medicine. In the process, we have changed the way we think about certain things and would like to pass on some energy-saving tips.

Concern about clothes is an incredible energy waster. Try to wear clothes that don't need ironing or special care. You should also consider using a laundry service if you can afford one. Some laundry services do a very good job and are not prohibitively expensive.

Cleaning the house is also very draining. We contacted a local church that had a program for helping the elderly and disabled. The people who take part in this program donate their services or charge a small fee. If you cannot find such a program, perhaps you could hire a high school student to help around the house.

Try to prepare simple meals. Find out if there is a Meals on Wheels program in your area. This program brings inexpensive meals right to your doorstep. There are also grocery stores and restaurants that will deliver food or meals.

Cleaning up after a meal can be more draining than preparing it. Consider investing in a dishwasher. If that is too expensive, try using as many paper products as you can. It is much easier to throw out a plate than it is to wash and dry it.

Save yourself from errands by shopping and banking by mail. When we do run errands, we organize them so we can accomplish them all during one outing. We limit using our car to only once or twice a week, forcing us to make better use of our time out. We have to rely on friends and relatives to help with household chores. For example, my parents help with grocery shopping and cooking, as well as taking care of some of our correspondence and phone calls.

We have learned to think of ourselves as a little cup full of life-sustaining water. Any activity, no matter how trivial, depletes this water. Since our illness prevents us from refilling the cup, it becomes our responsibility to guard the water as we would guard our life.

## COPING EMOTIONALLY

Understanding your illness entails not only learning how to change the way you think. You must also comprehend how CFS affects you emotionally. Every patient with CFS must learn to recognize and cope with many difficult emotions, especially anger, helplessness, loneliness, self-pity, guilt, discouragement, and fear. These emotions recur with distressing regularity. I want to share some of the painful emotions I struggle with, as well as some of the ways I try to cope with them.

## ANGER

I used to consider myself a very even-tempered person, slow to anger, slow to lash out. CFS has changed all that. I don't think my basically tranquil personality has been irrevocably altered, but it has undergone some incredible changes. A pool of anger boils and bubbles within me. Without warning, I can erupt like a volcano, incinerating the innocent in my fiery path.

Though CFS is the fundamental source of my anger, it is rarely the recipient. It cannot be scathed or tempered even by the most emotional outburst, therefore, I tend to pick out more vulnerable targets, like Shawn. My angry outbursts are usually triggered by someone or something causing me to expend my energy. Just as a scuba diver's life depends on conserving his oxygen, I must conserve my energy. I become angry when I am forced to waste my strength on inconsequential endeavors. Even something as trivial as being asked to repeat myself can ignite the flames of anger within me. When I am feeling very ill, the slightest irritation can generate the angriest outburst.

I struggle every day merely to survive. I feel as if I am precariously balanced on a tightrope, crossing a deep and deadly gorge. Every ounce of strength is needed just to keep my balance. I lash out in anger because I am afraid of falling. When my defenses are worn down and I feel threatened, my instincts take over. I attack before being attacked.

Frustration is a key component of anger, and my illness is a constant source of frustration. Each frustration that is ignored or denied festers, along with other suppressed frustrations. My anger can range from simple annoyance to vindictive outrage, but it usually burns itself out quickly. I find that the key to coping with anger successfully is releasing it. Don't suppress it. Anger is a natural and inevitable part of life. It is as normal an emotion as happiness; it just happens to be a lot louder.

In order to vent anger safely and healthily, it is important to identify the source of that anger. Obviously, CFS is the primary reason I am angry, but it is rarely the immediate cause. Anger may be caused by an insensitive friend who pretends to believe your illness is real but obviously has doubts. Or maybe you are expected to do something that is beyond your ability. Perhaps you are angry because you have been sick for so long. If you do not identify the triggering cause of your anger, you run the risk of misdirecting it. Inevitably, the target of misdirected anger will be the people who deserve it the least—you or your loved ones.

Try to be aware of your emotions, right from the first moment you start to feel angry. The old trick of counting to ten really does help. It gives you a chance to think about what you are doing before you react. If you are able, use that time to do an emotional self-evaluation. Look at the situation objectively. We often become needlessly angry because we think we have been wronged in some way, when in fact it is our perception that is wrong.

My wife has a loving and gentle spirit, and is always quick to consider the other person's point of view. That used to drive me crazy. I didn't want to see the other person's side or give him or her the benefit of the doubt. I wanted only to be mad! The more she taught me about the gracious art of compassionate understanding, however, the more I realized how truly rare righteous indignation is.

Some people internalize their anger, punishing themselves for their perceived failures. They often feel betrayed and abandoned by their own bodies so they seek to get even in the only way they know how: self-hatred. This is a form of emotional suicide and can be just as destructive. Another way we can hurt ourselves is by hurting those closest to us. We punish others in order to punish ourselves.

The tendency to lash out at others is greatly increased when we are very ill. We feel out of control and helpless. We may need to feel that we still have an impact on someone else's life, even if that impact is angry and hurtful, even if the people we hurt are people we love. Perhaps we have a hard time expressing our need for attention, so we grab it in any way we can. Or we may lash out in anger at our loved ones simply because we are afraid. We may be fearful that we are no longer lovable and that our loved ones may desert us. We hurt them because we fear they are going to hurt us. This can become a self-fulfilling prophecy: Our hurtful behavior ends up making us unlovable.

Once you become attuned to identifying the cause of your anger, you should try to avoid those situations that are most likely to make you angry. Many such situations are unavoidable, of course, but even they will be easier to deal with if you eliminate the ones you can. I have found that ignoring my own limitations is the greatest provocation of anger. When I push myself to the point of exhaustion, I no longer have the strength to control my anger.

Finally, learn to be forgiving, not only of others but of yourself as well. People are fallible; we all make mistakes. Share your feelings with those you love. If you are hurt by someone, talk it out. Don't hold grudges. A grudge doesn't hurt the person you are angry with; it only hurts you.

## HELPLESSNESS

It is not easy to be seen as helpless in a society that prides itself on its go-it-alone mentality. Rugged individualism, not helpless dependence, is respected and admired. The need for the help of others is often seen as a sign of weakness rather than acknowledged as a natural consequence of being human.

I don't have the option of blindly ignoring my humanness. My illness is a constant reminder of how terribly frail and vulnerable I am. Sometimes I am not even certain I can continue the fight, that I can endure bravely and stoically. And in our society, gold medals are given for winning the race, not for struggling to stay in it.

You may no longer be able to do the things you want or have the strength to do the things you need. If you have a severe case of CFS, you may be totally dependent on the help and support of others, physically, financially, and emotionally. It is a horrible feeling to be unable to take care of your basic needs. However, needing and being needed are as basic to humanity as breathing or eating, and do not make you any less of a person. Those who pride themselves on walking alone through life deprive themselves of one of the greatest joys of living.

You may also feel weak and helpless because you are unable to influence your recovery. But remember: Recovering from an illness requires no great feat of strength; your body is designed to do that naturally and unconsciously. What does require incredible inner strength is enduring a chronic illness. Helpless people do not endure chronic illness—they succumb to it.

You deserve admiration, not derision, for what you endure. Many people with CFS have humbly learned to endure a level of pain and sickness that would devastate a healthy person. Considering the cultural values we were all raised with, it takes a lot more strength and courage to ask others for help than it does to suffer silently—and needlessly—alone.


## LONELINESS

Loneliness may be the most prevalent emotional problem among Americans today, and this is especially true of people who suffer with CFS. I can be in a room full of people and feel totally alone, completely isolated by this illness. I often feel as if I am on the outside of life looking in, no longer sharing any common interests with the rest of society. Forced out of the world of health and activity, I have been dragged into a world of sickness and pain. I have joined a different brotherhood of humanity, the brotherhood of suffering.

It is natural to feel lonely when you are chronically ill. People with CFS can't help but feel different from most other people. The more intense this feeling, the more difficult it is to reach out to others. Your healthy friends may not visit anymore because they feel uncomfortable, not knowing what to say or what to do. You get tired of having to explain your illness all the time, and after a while it just seems easier to be alone.

To deal with loneliness, you must first decide that you don't want to be alone. I am not referring here to solitude. I love being alone when it is my choice. Loneliness is a feeling of total isolation. You may have physical proximity to other people, but no emotional closeness.

It is not easy reaching out to others when you are chronically ill. There is an inherent fear of rejection. You may fear that people won't accept you because you are ill, or even that they won't accept you because they don't believe you are ill. You must confront these fears head-on. Unfortunately, you cannot avoid meeting insensitive people, but you can't let them prevent you from reaching out to others.

One of the best ways to combat loneliness is meeting with other people who have CFS. You can derive comfort from the realization that you are not alone. There are thousands of people who have the same illness you do. I have been at support group meetings where new members burst into tears of relief because they had finally met someone who understood what they were going through.

Empathy counteracts loneliness. If there is no support group in your area, you can at least talk to someone with CFS over the phone. I have had many phone conversations with other CFS patients and while it is not as personal as meeting them, just talking seemed to help a lot. You can also meet with people who have other serious or chronic illnesses. Even though they may not know some of the specific trials you experience with CFS, they can still be empathetic and caring. My Aunt Kaye recently passed away, but for years she was one of my greatest sources of encouragement. She suffered from what seemed to be a lifetime of crippling rheumatoid arthritis, but her spirit was as gentle and loving as when she was well. In comparison to her suffering, my illness is minor, yet she never made me feel that way. She knew the agony of illness better than anyone, and the example of her life is my source of inspiration.

Finally, try to be the kind of person others enjoy being with. If you are continually angry or feeling sorry for yourself, no one is going to want to spend time with you. Try not to make other people feel guilty for being well. If you are envious of the health of your friends, you will drive them away. It is a safe bet that if you are the type of person others enjoy being with, you will not be lonely for very long.

## SELF-PITY

Self-pity is an emotion we are often unable to recognize within ourselves. It so warps our perceptions that we cannot look at ourselves objectively. Often we don't want to deal with this emotion because, in small doses, it makes us feel better. Initially, it even gains us sympathy from the people around us. But self-pity is like a drug; it may make us feel better temporarily, but the price we pay is too costly. People who feel sorry for themselves are miserable to be around. They are unable to care for anyone other than themselves, and soon there is no one left to care but themselves.

Isolated by your own self-involvement, you will see yourself as an undeserving victim. Your self-pity will intensify as each new perceived injustice leaves you feeling betrayed.

Eventually, people will think that you are doing such a good job generating sympathy on your own that you don't need any help. The sympathy you are so desperately trying to engender will never be given.

My greatest struggle against self-pity comes when I compare myself to other people. I feel as if they have everything in the world and I have nothing. All of our friends and relatives have purchased homes and cars. Not only have they had babies, but they are so far ahead of us they now have teenagers (all right, I don't envy everything)! Most are doing well in their jobs and all of them have more money than we do. Very soon I am feeling that their lives are totally fulfilling, and mine is totally empty. They are incredibly happy, while I am incredibly miserable.

When you are feeling sorry for yourself, you lose the ability to separate truth from projection. Sure, most of our friends have houses and children, and all of them have more money than we do. But their lives are not picture-perfect. They have problems of their own. Neither is my life totally void. I have a loving wife, caring friends, a supportive family, and a faithful Lord.

It is normal to feel sorry for yourself once in a while, but if you are not careful, self-pity could easily turn into resentment. Rather than sharing in the lives and successes of your friends and relatives, you could become envious and bitter, walking around with a chip on your shoulder. Thinking that you were somehow cheated in this life, you would blame everyone and everything for your misfortune. In short, you would become your own worst enemy, for these destructive attitudes would separate you from the love and support you so desperately need.

You may consider the old adage "Count your blessings" to be merely a cliché. Perhaps you feel that your blessings could be counted on one finger! If you are honest with yourself, though, you may be able to begin appreciating quite a few blessings in your life. It is very important for all of us to try to develop an attitude of thankfulness.

## GUILT

You cannot suffer the life-altering impact of CFS without also suffering feelings of guilt. It seems to be around every corner ready to pounce. Guilt comes from many different sources. You may feel guilty because you can no longer fulfill your obligations to your family, take proper care of the children, or bring home a paycheck. Whatever the circumstances, CFS prevents people from fulfilling many of their normal roles and obligations. This invariably leads to pangs of guilt.

You may even feel guilty due to the illness itself. You know you need to talk about your struggles, yet you may feel guilty doing so because CFS is not an illness that most people understand. You may not look severely ill, and you don't want to sound like a complainer. Or you may be wondering if you are somehow responsible for becoming ill. Perhaps you failed to take your health seriously enough, or didn't pay attention when your body was pleading with you for rest.

Whatever the reason, guilt is a destructive emotion that should not be regarded lightly. It eats away at you, making you feel weak, inadequate, and insecure. Guilt often stems from being too critical and unforgiving of yourself.

It helps to realize that the perceived source of guilt is usually unfounded. For example, you may feel guilty because you are unable to do the things you believe you are supposed to do. These feelings are based on unrealistic expectations of your health and, possibly, an unrealistic assessment of what others truly expect of you.

Share your feelings with those around you. You may be surprised to learn that you are the only one who expects so much of yourself. If others do expect more than you can give, they may be unaware of the severity of your illness. Don't assume that most people are sensitive enough to realize the true state of your health. I have found that I have to verbalize and demonstrate the severity of my affliction before people are able to understand.

Examine the source of your guilt. Try to determine if mistaken perceptions or unrealistic expectations are the actual source of the problem. If you find that the source of your guilt is other people, discuss it with them. They may be projecting their own feelings of inadequacy and guilt onto you.

Finally, do not be preoccupied with thoughts of retribution or punishment. Don't be obsessed with looking backward, trying to determine why you became ill. That doesn't matter now, and you need to spend your energy constructively in order to cope with this illness.

## DISCOURAGEMENT

Discouragement is often the result of the suppression of other emotions, such as guilt and anger. Often when CFS victims look back over the course of their illness and see how long they have been suffering—then look forward and find no relief in sight—a tidal wave of discouragement comes rushing over them, threatening to drown them in a sea of despair.

When I experience discouragement, I am able to see only the negatives in my life. Nothing is going right, and living is more a burden than a blessing. I am tired of being sick and sick of being tired. I am frustrated because I am unable to do the things I want and, more important, I am unable to be the type of person I want to be. Totally helpless and defeated by this disease, I have lost almost everything that is of value to me: my ability to work and provide for my family, my ability to be the husband Shawn deserves, my ability to have children, my freedom, my health, and my ability to serve God as a minister. I feel stretched to the absolute limits of my emotional and physical ability to endure. But just when I reach my breaking point, I discover something truly remarkable: an ability to endure beyond what I thought was my limit. This is not something I am quick to take credit for; I feel more like an astonished bystander watching this miraculous display.

This ability to survive is not unique to me. When you are overcome with discouragement and have reached the end of your endurance, encourage yourself that you can endure. Any limits you perceive are just that: perceived. There are no limits to your ability to endure. You can, and must, endure the trials of this illness.

Avoid making any major decisions when you feel this way. Discouragement is like a long, dark tunnel. You may not see the light at the end of the tunnel, but it is there. Be patient and you will soon be out of the darkness and into the light.

Learning to accept the limitations of your illness may help prevent discouragement. Don't be self-critical; rather, learn the art of self-loving and forgiving. People who have a hard time liking themselves fall more easily into the clutches of discouragement.

When you feel discouraged, reinforce positive behavior and change your environment or routine. Open the shades and let the sun shine in. Turn off the TV and go for a short walk, or sit outside breathing the fresh air. Listen to joyful or soothing music, or take a warm bubble bath. Maybe you should even consider getting a pet. Treat yourself by doing things that make you happy. Above all, reach out to others for help. Talk about your discouragement and vent your feelings with a good cry. Don't dwell on the past or worry about the future; just try to get through today. Finally, it is critical that discouragement not be allowed to build to the point of depression. Depression is an illness in its own right and once acquired may not be affected by attempts at changing your thoughts or attitudes.

## FEAR

It is understandable if CFS makes you anxious. Sometimes I am afraid to meet new people because I am self-conscious about my illness. Even though I have learned to expect them, I still dread the looks of doubt and disbelief. It is a universal human weakness to worry about what other people may think.

I am also afraid of the effects my illness may have on my body. No one knows the long-term effects of CFS. I wonder if I am more susceptible to other diseases, or whether this illness will make me weaker than I already am. I wonder if the medications I have taken will do more harm than good. I am afraid of the future—that I may never be well enough to have children or to complete my seminary training. Contemplating questions that have no easy answers invariably leads to worry and to fear. General feelings of apprehension and concern are a natural result of being chronically ill, but intense feelings of dread and paralyzing anxiety are not normal. You may feel afraid because you feel threatened and helpless, but you can't allow these feelings to ruin your life. You can't let your fear of people's disbelief prevent you from living. You can't let your fear of medications prevent you from trying safe treatments that might make you well. And you can't let your fears of the effects of your illness prevent you from living as well as you can with that illness.

If your biggest fear is that you may be developing some illness even more threatening than CFS, tell your physician. He or she can provide the testing necessary to reassure you of where you stand. If your anxiety is that you may be shunned by friends and colleagues who have heard through the grapevine that you are sick with some mysterious illness, the best thing you can do is talk openly with them. Explain what they need to know about CFS. Reassure them that they are in no danger.

Support groups are the best way I know to conquer anxiety. They allow you to express your fears and concerns to others who are dealing with those same feelings. Sharing and confronting fear is the best way I know to dispel it. But if, after sharing your feelings with your peers, you still feel overwhelmed with anxiety, I strongly urge you to seek professional help.

## COPING WITH YOUR SPIRITUAL NEEDS

I have received hundreds of letters from people all over the world in response to the first edition of this book. I was amazed at how many of them were seeking answers to spiritual questions. All too often, CFS delivers such a devastating blow that it literally rocks the very foundation of people's lives, leaving them wondering, Why is God allowing this to happen? Or, What is my purpose in life? If any of us are ever to find true peace amidst this suffering, we need to come to grips with the spiritual aspect of our lives.

I was studying to be a minister, and yet I too have wrestled with these same issues. CFS stripped away the veneer of everything I was supposed to believe and forced me to reaffirm the core issues of what I truly believe. Because of that I now have a deeper and more vital faith, based on a simple yet profound foundation; God loves me and I can trust him. I believe that we all have an innate need for God. It's as if there is an emptiness in our beings that only he can fill. Dealing with a chronic illness and the pain it inflicts merely intensifies our awareness of this. It is easier to ignore this void in our lives when we are healthy because the sense of frailty and transience that illness engenders is typically masked by the busy-ness and toil of everyday life.

I also believe that, despite my condition, God loves me and has a purpose for my life. I personally could not bear the thought of purposeless suffering, the belief that all the wrongs of this world are somehow meaningless acts of random misfortune. If God is not going to use my suffering for some higher good, then my suffering is in vain. But if, as God promises in the Bible, "all things work together for good for those who love him" (Romans 8:28), then I can find comfort in the knowledge that my illness is fulfilling some higher purpose. Does that mean I know what that purpose is? Not always. Like Job in the Old Testament, sometimes the reasons behind our suffering are not made known to us, but that doesn't make their impact any less significant. God sustained Job in the midst of his suffering, and his example served as a testimony in the heavenly realms to angel and demon alike.

God's compassion is beyond words and his comfort beyond description. I would not be able to survive this illness without him. His touch upon my life is what enables me to survive every day, and I know he has the same to offer any one of you. The Bible says that the Lord is "abounding in love to all who call upon him." If you would like to learn more about that love, please contact me through Warner Books.

I realize that all this "good advice" has only limited value to those of you who are too sick to act on it. I also know that when you are suffering, encouragement and advice often seem shallow and worthless. No matter what I write, or how much your family and friends may love you, you still face your pain alone. My only hope is that this chapter encourages you by showing that, while you suffer alone, you are not alone in your suffering. There are others who know what you are going through. I also recommend a book entitled *Finding Strength in Weakness,* by Lynn Vanderzalm. Lynn's family, as well as seventy CFS patients (including Shawn and I), shared thoughts and ideas on coping with CFS in this book.

Remember that there is no right way of coping with CFS. We all maintain our balance in different ways. My chief coping mechanism is limited avoidance. I put off dealing with things that I am unable to handle. This allows me to postpone until tomorrow what I am unable to face today.

Some people cope by denying their illness, while others are constantly concerned about it. At different times, you might need to use various coping mechanisms to learn what is effective in a given situation. Sometimes you may go with the flow, while other times you need to be contemplative and rational. At times you may deny and avoid your illness, and other times you may prefer to be actively involved. Sometimes you may feel like interacting with people, and other times you may need to withdraw. All you can do is take each hour one hour at a time. Do whatever is necessary to help you through that hour. If your illness is less severe than mine, coping may not be as difficult as I have depicted. If your illness is more severe, it may actually be more difficult. If you continue to have problems coping with CFS, seek professional help.

Finally, remember to weep when you need to weep, for a false sense of stoic strength only leads us to stiffen and break rather than soften and bend. And share your pain with others, for only a false sense of pride would cause us to insist on bearing this most terrible of burdens alone.

# CHAPTER EIGHT

# Overcoming Financial Hardship

*It took me a very long time to admit to myself that my illness
was not going to go away—that until such time as a cure was
discovered, I would be disabled. But eventually it became
painfully obvious that even the slightest activity made me feel
terribly ill and that continuing my education or holding down
a job was impossible.*

I still remember what I was feeling when I came to the realization that I needed Social Security disability benefits: hopelessness and shame. I felt hopeless because I was at the mercy of an
illness that was ruining me in every possible way, including
financially. I felt shame because I was brought up in a generation that looked down on people who accepted "handouts."
Even though I had been sick and unable to work for so long that
I really had no choice in the matter, it still did not make the
process any easier for me emotionally or psychologically.

Therefore, though I have been on disability, I understand
why the thought of receiving financial aid may be difficult for
some of you. Your self-esteem may be tied to your job or to how
much money you earn, making the prospect of being on disability, with a subsequent loss of income, too much to bear.
Maybe you resent the loss of self-sufficiency that receiving aid
implies. Perhaps accepting disability means admitting that you
are sick and can no longer hold on to your hopes and dreams;
you feel as if you are giving up and giving in to your illness.

Though I can empathize with those feelings, I would still

encourage you to consider applying for benefits if working is hurting your health. My hope is that you will avoid the mistake I made. My health deteriorated because I pushed myself to the breaking point, afraid to concede that I might not overcome my illness. Rather than think that you have no financial alternative but to work, at least consider the possibility that you may have no other "health" alternative but to stop.

For some of you, deciding whether to apply for Social Security benefits may not center around the difficulty of receiving financial help. Instead, the mere thought of applying for benefits may engender feelings of failure or surrender. Believe me, this is not the case. If any of us fell off a boat and were in danger of drowning we would all grasp for a life ring thrown to us. For the seriously ill, disability benefits can be received with gratitude rather than humiliation, if you realize that they give you the only chance you have of surviving your illness. It is no overstatement to assert that financial hardship presents one of the greatest health risks facing the chronically ill. That is because the fear of financial hardship can coerce the chronically ill to continue working at their jobs even though the strain of employment is literally making them ill. Often, quitting is never even considered because they mistakenly believe that they have no financial alternatives. But there *are* alternatives, and that is precisely the point of this chapter.

Now, unless you are independently wealthy (or no longer care about eating), you cannot just decide one day that you are no longer going to work. Since there is every chance you are going to be sick for quite some time, you have to make financial arrangements. For example, during the first few years of our illness, Shawn and I desperately needed Medicare to cover the expense of treatments, which ran into tens of thousands of dollars. Our families didn't have that kind of money, so we followed the only logical course left open to us: We applied for disability benefits.

We live in a wonderful country that has emergency provisions for people in need. For years, your tax dollars have been hard at work providing for others who are less fortunate than yourself. These same dollars have also been set aside, in the form of Social Security and many other programs, against the event that you should ever become disabled.

I know that the prospect of taking government aid is often distasteful. Some of you may hold the misconception that any government program is a form of charity. It isn't! Social Security can be thought of as a type of insurance policy that you and your family have contributed to over your entire lifetimes. By paying Social Security and other taxes, you have provided not only for help during your retirement, but for times of hardship as well.

My father-in-law calculated that if he had taken all the Social Security taxes he has paid to the government and invested them wisely over the past thirty years, he would be able to support my wife and me with thousands of dollars a month for the rest of our lives. The sweat and hard labor that go into paying taxes entitle you to receive benefits. You wouldn't consider disability benefits from a private insurance company to be charity. In a very real sense, the government is just the largest insurer in the country.

We are blessed that we live in such a compassionate and caring country that makes provisions for the chronically ill. Applying for benefits may be a difficult choice, but it has been a lifesaver for many. It could be the right decision for you as well. I can't promise that you won't have to make some sacrifices, or even that once you quit your job you are assured of receiving benefits. However, if I have learned one fundamental truth from this illness, it is that there is nothing on this earth as precious as your health. Without it, you are unable to function on any level: spiritually, socially, emotionally, mentally, or physically. You need to guard it as jealously as you do your life, for if you ruin your health by pushing yourself unwisely, you run the risk of wasting your life.

The only factor, then, that should determine whether you apply for disability benefits is the extent of your disability. I won't pretend that the application process is easy, but by explaining the major programs, and by guiding you through some of the problems you might encounter in applying, I hope to make the process as painless as possible.

## EMPLOYEE BENEFITS

The very first step you should take is to speak with your employer and find out if your company provides disability benefits. Frequently companies do offer disability insurance for their employees, and these benefits are typically much easier to obtain than Social Security. Your personnel director or supervisor can explain how to apply.

## SOCIAL SECURITY

If your company has no disability provisions, you should contact the Social Security Administration office to apply for benefits. Never assume, for any reason, that you are ineligible. I was told by a hospital social worker that I was not entitled to benefits because I was a student and because my illness was not considered disabling. Fortunately, I have a persistent spirit and I refused to believe there wasn't some form of government aid to help people in my situation.

### ELIGIBILITY REQUIREMENTS

There are only two requirements you must meet in order to receive disability benefits. The first is that you be totally disabled, unable to perform even sedentary work. The second is that you have paid some Social Security taxes five out of the last ten years. This is a general rule, and there are exceptions. Call or go to your local Social Security office for more details. Students may also be eligible, because Social Security taxes were probably withheld from their salaries during summer employment.

Eligibility for disability benefits is not based on your income or assets. If, for some reason, you do not meet the two requirements, do not despair. You may still be eligible for financial aid in the form of welfare assistance, rental subsidy programs, Medicaid, or food stamps. These programs are discussed later in this chapter.

## YOUR FIRST VISIT

When you contact the Social Security office, you will be assigned a caseworker. The caseworker will have a record of your work history as well as a record of the amount you have paid in Social Security taxes. You must make sure that their records are correct because the amount of your monthly benefits depends in part on the amount of taxes you have paid.

Once you have determined that you have paid Social Security taxes and are eligible to apply, the next step is proving that you are disabled. Unfortunately, this is not the easiest of tasks. Unlike our judicial system, where you are considered innocent until proven guilty, at Social Security you are assumed to be able to work. It is up to you to prove you are not. If you are aware of this in advance, you will not be as easily discouraged if you are rejected and have to appeal. If you are patient and persistent, there is every likelihood that, in the end, you will be approved. Your caseworker will explain what you must do to file your initial application. It was my good fortune to have a caring and concerned caseworker who did not make me feel like a second-class citizen. But I have run into caseworkers who couldn't care less about me or my illness. Don't be intimidated by heartless caseworkers. Fortunately, they are not the people who decide your case.

Discussing your disability with a stranger can be embarrassing, especially since people with CFS often look so much better than they feel. Don't minimize the extent of your illness or the traumatic impact it has on your life just because you are afraid of sounding like a complainer. The only way Social Security can make a fair decision is if you let them have all the facts. When you are asked questions about your physical limitations, answer according to a typical day, not one of your better ones. Don't forget the particularly horrible days when you feel absolutely wretched. Explain your disability to the caseworker patiently and accurately. Don't exaggerate, but don't minimize.

Wading through this sea of bureaucratic red tape may make the Social Security system seem designed to be as discouraging as possible. Perhaps this is in response to all the attention that has recently been focused on the minority of people who abuse the system.

Whatever the reason, I don't think applying for Social Security has always been this intimidating. This change in attitude can be seen by comparing the old and new Social Security cards. My card, issued in the late sixties, politely informs me what to do should I ever lose my card or change my name. It says that when I reach age sixty-two, or if I am ever unable to work because of a disability, I should contact my local Social Security office. It even encourages me to inquire about retirement checks. To top it off, it invites me to sign up for Medicare when I reach sixty-two, even if I am not yet ready to retire. You get the impression that they really do want to help.

That's not the feeling you get reading my wife's Social Security card, which is much newer because her name changed when we were married. First comes a warning: "Do not laminate this card!" Then it says that the card is invalid if it is not signed. It proceeds to threaten her, saying that if she uses the card improperly she can be thrown in prison and fined. She is then reminded that the card is the property of the Social Security Administration and must be returned to them whenever they request it. Finally, at the very bottom of the card, they get around to the reason she even has it in the first place. They inform her that she should contact Social Security for any other matter. Are they kidding? After all that, I'd be afraid even to touch their card, let alone contact one of their offices!

All kidding aside, if you are prepared for the frustration of a long and difficult process, you will not be one of the people discouraged from receiving their benefits. In the end, when all the paperwork is finished, the system does provide for those who persevere. But you must be prepared for an incredibly invasive investigation. By the time they're finished, it will seem as if Social Security knows everything there is to know about you and a little more. From your finances to your medical records, they will leave no stone unturned.

## THE INITIAL APPLICATION

When you file your initial application, you will be asked many different questions, even some that seem to have no bearing on your illness. You will be asked how much you can lift, how far you can walk, how long you can sit, and so on. You will also be asked about the nature of your disability and why you are unable to work.

When answering these questions, be as specific as possible. Don't just tell them that you have chronic fatigue syndrome and expect them to understand. Tell them the ins and outs of your illness. You must prove not only that you are unable to perform your previous job, but that you are unable to perform any job, including sedentary labor. If you are completely disabled by your illness, explain that you can't walk, sit, or stand except for brief periods. Discuss your fatigue, your aches and pains, your mental impairment, and how you are affected when you try to work. Tell them how difficult it is just trying to do the chores around the house, how even the simple tasks of personal hygiene are draining.

## MEDICAL DOCUMENTATION

You will be asked to provide all your medical records, as well as specific medical evidence to support your claim. Social Security will contact your doctors directly to obtain their opinion of your disability. Do not assume that a simple statement that you are disabled will be enough to win your case. You need letters from your doctors that explain clearly and specifically why you are unable to do any type of work.

The letter below is not the one I used when I applied, but it is much like the one I would use today. Show it to your doctors to use as a guide, though of course some of the specifics mentioned, for example treatment with gamma globulin, may not apply to every patient. Your letter(s) should be tailored to your specific circumstances.

> Social Security Administration
> Bureau of Disability Determination
>
> To Whom It May Concern:
>
> I am writing to certify that Jane Doe is completely disabled for performance of even sedentary tasks due to the following debilitating conditions.
> Jane Doe has been suffering the effects of chronic fatigue syndrome, and mild hypogammaglobulinemia. She has undergone detailed sophisticated medical, immunologic, and physical examinations, which, along with my long-term treatment of the patient, since March 1995, constitute the basis for my professional conclusions.

Individuals so infected as Ms. Doe have severely disabling symptoms of fatigue, malaise, recurrent pharyngitis, cervical and inguinal adenopathy, arthralgia, lethargy, weakness, and low-grade fever. She is also seriously debilitated by the following neurological symptoms: dizziness, headaches, mental fogging, confusion, and an inability to think clearly or concentrate. These symptoms have persisted since their onset in February 1994 and, due to the degree of their severity, have rendered her totally disabled.

Following the diagnostic guidelines for chronic fatigue syndrome established by Fukada, et al. in the December 15, 1994 *Annals of Internal Medicine,* Ms. Doe exhibits all the classic symptoms used to diagnose this syndrome. She has also undergone sophisticated tests to rule out any other possible diseases. She has undergone immunoglobulin subclass tests, which reveal partial immunoglobulin deficiency. Physical examinations reveal shotty nodes in the posterior cervical and inguinal areas.

Ms. Doe's historical, clinical, serologic, and immunologic findings are entirely consistent with the diagnosis of chronic fatigue syndrome.

In the summer of 1995, Ms. Doe began receiving intravenous gamma globulin treatments for her immune deficiency. Other empiric trials include acyclovir, Diamox, Pamelor, Sinequan, Nardil, and vitamin therapy, all without significant or sustained benefits. She has also tried alternative therapies such as acupuncture, homeopathy, chiropractic care, and special diets without improvement.

Jane Doe is capable of standing, walking, carrying, lifting, and doing sedentary tasks while sitting down only sporadically or for an insignificant amount of time. She needs to rest between activities. Jane Doe is unable to perform even a sedentary job part time. Chronic fatigue syndrome has severely limited both her physical and

mental capacity to perform even basic activities. Her neurological symptoms render any activity requiring concentration, including reading and driving, very difficult. She
is capable of only mild activity on an intermittent basis.
Most days, she may be able to do no more than wash,
dress, and prepare meals. On other days, she may be able
to take care of correspondence or do some light reading.
Her ability to sustain any activity for more than a few
hours a day is unpredictable, and any prolonged activity
(even sedentary activity) worsens her condition and could
cause exacerbation of her symptoms.

Ms. Doe has unsuccessfully attempted low-stress
activities many times, but, as for most people with this
syndrome, any activity results in a worsening of her
symptoms. Restricting activity is, at present, the only
way to prevent exacerbation of the symptoms.

I have had experience in evaluating and treating
many patients with CFS. The fatigue these patients suffer with is unlike the normal fatigue experienced by
healthy individuals. It is a profound weakness that
makes simple tasks such as brushing their teeth seem
overwhelming. Although individuals with this syndrome
frequently do not appear significantly ill, most are, in
fact, markedly disabled and are frequently unable to be
gainfully employed.

Patients are typically young or middle-aged adults
who fail to fully recover clinically and immunologically
from this syndrome. Detailed observations have been
reported by Fukada, et al. in "The Chronic Fatigue
Syndrome: A Comprehensive Approach to Its Definition
and Study" (*Annals of Internal Medicine,* 1994;
121:953–959).

In conclusion, I do not know whether Jane Doe's disability is likely to resolve. Very few chronic fatigue syndrome patients have experienced spontaneous improvement. There is no known cure or medication that is
effective in treating this syndrome, and since Ms. Doe

has not experienced any relief from the best available therapies, it is my opinion that she will continue to be disabled and unable to be employed in any manner for an indeterminate period of time.

I will be following Jane Doe in the near future and will continue other forms of investigational therapy to counteract the ravages of chronic fatigue syndrome.

If I can be of further help in the support of Jane Doe's application for disability benefits, please don't hesitate to call on me.

Sincerely,

M. J. Leavay, M.D.

Any letters your doctors write should attempt to be as detailed and specific as the one above. They must stress that you are unable to do any type of work, including sedentary tasks, and the reasons why (for example, that activity worsens your condition). It should also explain the nature of your illness as well as your symptoms, and should validate the severity of your illness, especially regarding the limitations it imposes. Social Security will acknowledge your limitations only if they are validated by a doctor. If your doctor can prove that you have other ailments as well as CFS, your chances of being accepted may be improved. For example, you might also be diagnosed with an immune deficiency, sleep disorders, fibromyalgia, or neurally mediated hypotension.

If you have more than one doctor, have each of them write a letter. Since doctors' letters are one of the most important ways you have of proving you are disabled, it is important that you keep seeing your doctors regularly. Notify them that they will soon be contacted by Social Security. Any delay on their part in sending your records or writing their opinions slows down the process.

At this point, you have the option of informing your senators or congressmen that you have applied for Social Security. They have no influence to help you win your case, but they will let the Social Security office know they are interested in the results of your application. At the very least, this special interest should help keep your claim from being delayed or getting lost. In other words, Social Security is being held accountable by an elected official.

After your initial application is finally done, your medical evidence submitted, and your representatives contacted, all that is left to do is wait for Social Security's decision. This will take weeks or even months. When that fateful day does arrive, do not be discouraged if your initial application is rejected. Social Security does now recognize CFS as a legitimate disabling condition, but proving you have CFS and that you are disabled is not always easy. Social Security forwarded my first rejection to the National Institutes of Health, where I was having experimental drugs pumped into my veins in an effort to overcome this illness. It didn't seem to matter to Social Security that this was obviously the action of someone who was truly ill.

## THE FIRST APPEAL

If you are rejected, the second stage of your disability application is the appeal for reconsideration. This is very similar to the first stage. You have to fill out more forms and submit additional evidence to support your claim. The person who decides your case at this point still has very strict guidelines to follow, but does have more flexibility. In other words, he or she can be more lenient when making the determination.

The chances of being approved for chronic fatigue syndrome during the first two applications have increased dramatically since I first became ill, but do not be discouraged if you are once again rejected. You can appeal this rejection as well.

When I applied, this syndrome was totally unknown, and I knew that in all likelihood I would be rejected. Therefore, though it may now seem overly pessimistic, I regarded the initial application, as well as the appeal for reconsideration, as something to be dispensed with quickly. The sooner I could get this over with, I felt, the sooner I could move on to the second appeal—the appeal that made a difference.

## THE SECOND APPEAL

This second appeal is decided by an administrative law judge. Pleading your cause before a judge sounds more ominous than it is. Your hearing is not held in a court, but in an office. This hearing is where you make or break your case. Since it is such an important meeting, I recommend that you retain an attorney. It is a sad commentary on our society that the disabled and needy have to hire a lawyer just to secure what is rightfully theirs. For some reason, however, your chances of winning are increased when you hire a lawyer.

Make sure that you retain a lawyer who has experience with Social Security hearings. They typically work for a percentage of the retroactive benefits you receive if you win your case. Retroactive benefits are the accumulated monthly benefits you would have received all along had your initial application been accepted. If you were disabled for at least a year prior to filing your initial application, you may also be entitled to benefits for some of the months before you applied. Your Social Security caseworker can explain all the rules and requirements as well as calculate the retroactive benefits you are entitled to. If you cannot afford to pay an attorney a percentage of your retroactive benefits, you should contact your Social Security office or the local Legal Aid Society. They may know of lawyers who donate their services.

If one of your doctors is able to attend the hearing, your

chances of winning could be greatly increased. Your doctor's presence will have greater influence than a letter alone. If your doctor is kind enough to support you in this way, remember to compensate him or her. Our doctor, Dr. Oleske, was so kind he wouldn't even send us a bill, so we gave him a briefcase to thank him for his support.

The administrative law judge will ask you many questions. The following list contains some of the questions most frequently asked:

1. You will be asked to give your age, height, and weight and to tell if you are right-handed or left-handed.
2. You will be asked about your marital status, educational background, military record, and any special vocational training you have had.
3. You will be asked about your last job and how much lifting and bending it required. You will also be asked about the last day you worked and what prevented you from returning to work.
4. You will be asked if you can dress and feed yourself, as well as about any impairments you might have. You will be asked if you can perform housework, cooking, laundry, and shopping activities.
5. You will be asked how far you can walk and run, if you can touch the floor with your hands, and how long you can sit and stand comfortably.
6. You will be asked if you are able to drive a car, and, if not, how you got to the hearing.
7. You will be asked about your social contacts: if you visit friends, attend church, have any hobbies, or belong to any clubs or organizations.
8. You will be asked about your typical day: what time you get up, if you watch TV, and how much you sleep.
9. You may be asked about future vocational training, and a vocational expert may be called in to determine if you

can be trained to perform some job other than the one you had.

10. You will be asked about your aches and pains. You will be asked to explain, in your own words, how your illness prevents you from working. You will also be asked to describe any medications or treatments you are taking or have tried.

11. On a scale of one to ten, you will be asked to describe the level of pain you experience with and without medication. You will be asked how often you see a doctor.

12. Finally, you will be allowed to tell the judge anything that wasn't already covered regarding your illness.

This list of questions may seem intimidating, but try not to be afraid. Think about your answers. During the hearing, answer all the questions clearly and carefully. Once again, don't minimize your illness. The judge needs to know exactly what you are going through. Finally, try not to be too nervous. The majority of people I know who have applied for disability benefits have won. As CFS becomes more readily accepted, benefits should also become easier to obtain.

## THE APPEALS COUNCIL

There is a council, called the Appeals Council, that has the final say on all Social Security claims. This means that they have the power not only to grant you benefits even if the administrative law judge denies them, but also to deny your claim even if the administrative law judge approved it. They might do the former if they feel that the law judge was unfair in deciding your case, and they might do the latter if they feel he was not critical enough. It is unusual, however, for the Appeals Council to overturn a favorable decision.

If you are denied benefits, it will probably mean one of two things: Either you are not totally disabled, or you have not presented strong enough medical evidence to prove your case. If the administrative law judge denies your claim, you can request that your case be heard by the Appeals Council. Make sure you give them conclusive evidence of your disability, with very supportive doctors' letters. If it was the Appeals Council that denied your claim, your case will probably be sent back to the administrative law judge for review. In this case, the same advice applies: Submit strong, conclusive evidence and doctors' letters. If after all this you are still denied, and you firmly believe you are disabled, you have only two recourses. One is to file a lawsuit, and the other is to repeat the entire process all over again—not an appealing prospect, but it just might work.

Just a few loose ends to tie up before ending this section on obtaining Social Security benefits: Don't put off applying. The date you file is very important. Your retroactive disability benefits only date back a maximum of one year before your filing date, regardless of how long you have been disabled. If you are too ill to apply in person, an application can be sent to you in the mail, or you may appoint a close friend or family member to be your representative. My parents spent many hours at the Social Security office helping me obtain my benefits.

If you are awarded benefits, you will also be eligible for Medicare, which is a reasonable health insurance plan for the disabled and elderly. It pays 80 percent of approved doctors' fees. You are not eligible, however, until two years after you first become disabled and one year after your filing date.

## SUPPLEMENTAL SECURITY INCOME

For those of you who are disabled but have not worked long enough to be eligible for disability benefits, or for those of you who are eligible for benefits but whose monthly payments are not enough to keep you above the federally mandated poverty level, there is a program available to help. It is called Supplemental Security Income (SSI), a form of welfare that is administered through Social Security. Age is not a factor for this program; children as well as adults are eligible as long as their income is low. Since welfare programs are partially financed by the states, each state has its own rules and regulations.

Applying for SSI is similar to applying for disability benefits. If you can prove you are disabled and your income and your assets are within the guidelines, then you are eligible for SSI. Your income is the amount of money you receive each month from any source, such as disability benefits, stock dividends, money from friends and relatives, and so on. Sometimes things you receive in place of money, such as food and shelter, are also counted as income. (Children living at home and not paying for food and housing will have some of their parents' assets and income counted.) Assets are things you own, such as stocks, bonds, savings and checking accounts, real estate, and some personal property. Your home is not counted as an asset. Your automobile as well as some personal possessions, depending on their value, may not be counted either. Social Security will inform you what is considered an asset and what is not.

If you think you might be eligible for SSI, it is easiest to apply for it at the same time you apply for disability benefits. You will be asked to fill out many forms and answer many questions. Bring with you proof of your income and assets, such as payroll stubs, insurance policies, bankbooks, and checking account statements. Once it is determined that you are disabled and eligible for disability benefits, Social Security will compute your monthly earnings to see if you are eligible for SSI as well. SSI payments are typically much less than disability payments, and the amount differs from state to state. But the benefits are worth it if your disability benefits are not very high, or if you are disabled but have not worked enough to be eligible for Social Security disability.

# MEDICAID

In addition to monthly checks, SSI recipients are eligible to receive Medicaid, a free health insurance plan for people with low income. Medicaid is also available to people with other sources of income, so long as that income is low enough to qualify. Medicaid pays 100 percent of approved doctors' fees. Unfortunately, Medicaid typically does not approve the total amount that most doctors charge, so some doctors will not treat Medicaid patients. You may have to shop around a little to find a doctor who will.

# HOUSING ASSISTANCE

SSI recipients and others with low income may also be eligible for rental subsidy programs. The state, county, or even some townships may have housing subsidy programs for the elderly, disabled, and low-income families. Some programs have low-rent housing units available. Others, such as the Section 8 rental subsidy program, may require you to find your own apartment or house. With either type of program, you are responsible for paying approximately 30 percent of your income in rent; the government pays the remainder. You should contact your local Social Security office, county welfare agency, or hospital social worker to see if there are any programs available in your area.

Applying for rental subsidy is the same as applying for any government program—more forms and more questions. When applying, bring all your Social Security records proving your disability and any financial information you have. As with SSI, the amount of benefits you receive from these programs is dependent on your income and assets.

## FOOD STAMPS

SSI recipients and others with low income may also be eligible for food stamps. As with rental subsidy, you usually apply for food stamps at a different agency than Social Security, but Social Security can inform you where that agency is located. Again, you will have lots of forms to fill out and lots of questions to answer. And as with any of these programs, eligibility is dependent on your income and your assets. If you are eligible for food stamps, you are given a special card, like a credit card, that allows you to receive food stamps from most grocery stores. You take this card with you when you go shopping, and the grocery store runs it through a computer to see what amount you are entitled to. (Actually, "stamps" is a misnomer. What you receive is a booklet filled with coupons of different denominations.) You then use these stamps at the grocery store the same way you would use cash. However, food stamps cannot be used for all grocery items, only for food products.

## PERIODIC REVIEW

Once you've been approved for any of the above programs, including disability benefits, you are subject to periodic review. It may be done as frequently as once each year, or it might not happen for three or four years, but eventually Social Security and the other agencies will get around to reviewing your case. This process is typically the same as when you first applied. For disability benefits, you will need medical evidence and strong doctors' letters to prove that you are still disabled. If you applied for SSI, or any welfare programs, you will have to prove that your income and assets have not changed substantially.

If your benefits are discontinued as a result of a review, you can request a hearing for reconsideration. This basically follows the same procedure as when you first applied. For disability, your case will be reviewed by an administrative law judge. Don't be discouraged if you have to go through this process. If you are truly disabled or in need of financial help, you have a very good chance of having your benefits reinstated.

In closing, please remember that there is financial help available, and for many of you, it would be worth your while to make the effort to obtain it. Disability benefits and other forms of assistance give you options, and options make coping with this illness a whole lot easier.

# CHAPTER NINE

# Advice for Family and Friends

*Caring for someone who is chronically ill is a labor of love. It is a labor because it is an arduous struggle with a disease whose demands are not limited to weeks, but to years. But the harshness of this labor is tempered by the mellifluence of love. The endeavor shines forth as a wonderful example of love's purest form: self-sacrifice.*

I never cease to be amazed at how crucial the understanding and support of those close to me remains. To me, there is nothing more healing than being loved and accepted by one's family and friends. I find that I no longer greatly fear the doubts or derision of strangers because the people that matter the most to me have no such doubts. They have an unshakable belief in the validity of my affliction and it gives me an inner strength that is not easily broken.

Having the rather unique distinction of not only being ill myself but caring for someone who is chronically ill, I also recognize the immense challenge that being a caregiver presents. I understand the many trials a whole family suffers when one of their own is hurting, for illness does not only affect the person it infects. The enormous problems caused by chronic fatigue syndrome can splinter even the closest of relationships, which is why I felt it important to include this chapter for family and friends.

Where do we find the strength to be a caregiver, to give so completely of ourselves? There is no genetic trait passed down over the generations that predisposes some to achieving this most noble of goals and others to failure. If it were as automat-ic as that, we would not esteem self-sacrificial love so highly. Selflessness is valued because it must be striven for.

Hardships require of us our excellence, but what is required is not beyond our grasp. If truth be told, none of us would choose to endure hardships of any kind, especially the hardships associated with illness. Choosing which is our por-tion to suffer, however, is a luxury we rarely enjoy. In this regard, loving and caring for someone who is chronically ill is the same as *being* chronically ill: You have no choice but to endure. Like ships foundering in a sudden storm, we brave the gales not because we want to, but because we have to. Often our finest moments are born not out of desire, but out of necessity.

There are countless times I would gladly have taken upon myself the pain of Shawn's illness—not solely for altruistic rea-sons, as many would suppose, but because to relieve her pain would relieve my own: Watching Shawn suffer hurt me more than words can express. Though my defenses could withstand the raging fury of my own illness, they were helpless against even the slightest whisper of Shawn's. I am sure that for many of you, the pain of loving someone but being unable to effect his or her cure may seem almost unbearable. Through years of weaving close personal relationships, a fabric of concern entwines people with those who love them. If you are a spouse, parent, child, or friend of someone with CFS, many of your hopes and aspirations may be inextricably intertwined with those of your loved ones. When their dreams are shattered, so are yours.

The responsibility of caring for someone with CFS may have been placed squarely on your shoulders. Initially, you may have accepted this burden willingly, but have now found it dif-ficult to bear as the months stretch into years. Sacrifices are eas-ier to start than to sustain. If your loved one were acutely and temporarily ill, the challenge would not be as great. We would all prefer the satisfaction of being lifesavers to the prosaic endurance of being life-sustainers.

In contrast to the respect and admiration accorded those who care for the acutely ill, caring for the chronically ill is done in relative obscurity. This is because, to outsiders, there is nothing inspiring or triumphant about chronic illness. Everything associated with the term *chronic* has negative connotations. You never hear anyone claiming to be chronically happy or chronically in love. The only time you hear the word *chronic* is in relation to unceasing illness.

It is just that sense of endlessness, the inability to derive strength from knowing your trials will soon be over, that can make the future seem terribly discouraging. This is not just a temporary commitment; it demands a total readjustment of the family structure and responsibilities.

## OVERCOMING RESENTMENT

Because of the continuous disruption this illness can cause in your lives, family members might harbor feelings of resentment at one time or another. This is quite understandable. The needs seem endless. No matter how much you do, it never seems to be enough. Feelings of frustration and irritability surface because you're overwhelmed by all that's required of you every day. Everything you planned for your lives may now seem hopelessly out of reach.

Countless problems and emotions must be dealt with each and every day. Your children may be having a hard time at school because they have a sibling or parent who is "different." You may even be losing some of your close friends because they don't understand this illness and are afraid it is contagious. Whatever the problem, it is important that you not neglect your own needs or the needs of the rest of your family. Everyone's emotional and physical strength must be kept up.

Because your loved one is at home sick, you may feel guilty when you spend time out enjoying yourself. You must remember, however, that your emotions need feeding as surely as your body does. Suppressing your own needs and feelings is unhealthy, and results in resentment, bitterness, and withdrawal. Then you will be caring for your loved one not out of love, but because you feel it is your responsibility. This can't help but be perceived, and will create barriers as strong as any erected by this illness.

## SHARING YOUR FEELINGS

One of the most important pieces of advice I can give any friend or family member affected by CFS is to rely on the help of others. When our CFS support group first began, I imagined its sole purpose would be to help those of us with this illness cope with our affliction. I never dreamed it would also serve as a place where family and friends could find comfort and understanding.

It was wonderful to see their needs being met in ways we never envisioned. They were comforted by the realization that they were not alone, that there were others who understood the heartrending trials of caring for someone with CFS. You need to be honest about your feelings and share them with someone who cares, if not at a support group, then with a close friend or relative, or perhaps even a counselor. We all need support and understanding to cope with this traumatic illness. It is not a sign of weakness but a sign of strength to go to others for help.

Don't be afraid to include your loved one among the people you go to for help. When Shawn and I first became ill, I made the foolish mistake of keeping most of my emotions locked away, deep inside. I felt guilty burdening Shawn with them; it seemed selfish to ask her to help me. I hoped that if I ignored my feelings, the problems and resentments would just go away. But suppressed emotions don't go away; they fester and grow.

I have since learned the importance of being honest with Shawn. It does neither of us any good to hide our true feelings from each other. Relationships are based on sharing. They require trust, and trust is built on honesty. If problems are concealed, your loved one will come to feel isolated and unneeded. The two of you may drift apart. In the end you may have two people with resentments: the caregiver, trapped with pent-up emotions, and the person with CFS, feeling untrustworthy and excluded from your life.

Of course, I try to be sensitive to Shawn's illness and not overwhelm her by expressing everything I am feeling at one time, but I don't deny my feelings in order to protect her. A balance must be achieved. If either of us is too ill to discuss something, we tell the other and save it for a day when we feel stronger.

## UNDERSTANDING YOUR LOVED ONE'S NEEDS

As you are no doubt aware, the changes wrought by CFS can make your loved one's life feel painfully out of control. Discouragement comes easily when treatments don't work, and pangs of guilt are an all-too-common companion when he or she realizes the effect of CFS on family and friends. All the things that used to make life worth living—job, self-esteem, even simple pleasures—may no longer seem relevant. I make these points because it is important that you understand that people who suffer with chronic illness have emotional, social, and spiritual needs, not just physical ones. You may be your loved one's only source of encouragement and support, so you need to be sensitive to all of these needs.

## PRESERVING INDEPENDENCE

One emotional need common to people with CFS is the need to feel independent. When someone else does all their cooking and cleaning, perhaps even makes many of their decisions, it is easy for CFS sufferers to become dependent on other people and lose their identity as adults. People with CFS need to be treated as adults and not children. Nothing should be hidden from them, because they will see right through it. Try not to be overprotective or smothering, and respect your loved one's privacy as well.

Family members should trust the judgment of their loved ones in regard to their limitations. People with CFS should never be pressured into activities they are not well enough to do. On the other hand, at times they may choose to be active in order to keep their spirits up. Express your concerns, but then allow your loved one to make the decision without imposing guilt. People with CFS are the only ones who can determine their limitations. You should also try to be supportive of any treatments that are undertaken, even if you have reservations. Your loved one must have the freedom to make the final decision.

Remember to think of the chronically ill as people and not patients. Be sensitive to their limitations, but don't define them by their CFS. Your loved one is no less a person because of this illness. Many people with CFS feel useless and superfluous. They need to have family and friends share their lives with them, allowing them to feel accepted and attached. People with CFS still need to feel important, so continue to go to them for advice or help. This allows them the opportunity to contribute to the family. Your loved ones need to know that you value them not just for what they do, but for who they are.

## ACCEPTANCE AND UNDERSTANDING

Another very important emotional need is to feel accepted and understood. You can help with this by acknowledging the hurt your loved one is experiencing and by expressing your concern and support. Acknowledging pain is as simple as saying, "I am so sorry that you are hurting. It hurts me to see you struggling. I want you to know that I will always be here for you if you need me." Don't belittle your loved one's pain by giving pat answers like, "Don't worry, you'll be well soon," or "At least your illness isn't fatal." If you don't acknowledge the severity of this affliction, your loved one will feel isolated and alone. Learn to listen, not only to what is said, but to what is meant. Many people say they are okay but really mean they are hurting.

Unfortunately, I have met family members who have a snap-out-of-it mentality about chronic illness. They delude themselves into thinking they are offering support and encouragement when they push and prod their loved one to act healthy. In reality, they are doing nothing but venting their impatience and frustration on an innocent victim. Before we were married, Shawn and I lived with our families. They bore the brunt of our depression and irritability, which are the hallmarks of this illness, as well as taking care of our daily physical and financial needs. Never once did either of our families make us feel guilty for being unable to be well. Their encouragement always took the form of, "It's all right that you're ill," rather than "I can't believe you're still ill."

## BE REALISTIC—BUT NOT NEGATIVE

Acknowledging pain is not the same as constantly dwelling on the illness, always emphasizing the negative. Be aware of what you say and how you treat someone with CFS. I have met families who continually say that their loved one's life is passing by, that his or her potential is being wasted. They constantly bring up the fact that their loved one is missing out on the best years of life and will never be able to relive them. This type of negative communication can be crippling.

The chronically ill measure their lives in months, not minutes. Healthy people run their lives by the clock: 45 minutes to get ready in the morning, 15-minute coffee break, 30 minutes for lunch, 25 minutes to drive home from work. If I thought of my life as minutes slipping by, I would not be able to cope with this illness another day.

My world is regulated not by the clock, but by the calendar. When I first became ill, I felt time rushing by faster than I could measure. Every day I was ill was a further postponement of my life. All my friends and relatives seemed to be passing me by.

It took me years to unlearn a healthy man's time reference, but I have finally succeeded. I no longer measure time from the beginning of my life, but from the end. I no longer look backward to see how many years have passed, but take hope by looking forward to how many years remain.

People with CFS already feel that in many ways they are waiting to live. They don't need to be constantly reminded of it. Without minimizing the illness, you should try to stress the positive. Try to make your loved one's life as normal and as enjoyable as possible.

## RUNNING INTERFERENCE

Your loved one's social needs are also very important. But one thing that can stand in the way of social pleasure is the insensitive remarks of other people. This is a place where you, as a concerned friend or relative, can help by being a social go-between. Perhaps a few examples of the situations I've faced will show you what I mean.

I found it very discomforting to answer probing questions about my illness. It can make me feel like an oddity at a circus sideshow. I don't believe that people who ask me probing questions are purposely trying to be cruel. They just don't realize how much pain their insensitive questions can inflict.

Then there are the incredulous comments: "You look so well!" More often than not the sentiment is well intentioned, but those four little words never encourage me; they make me feel stupid. I never know what to reply. I usually say that I try hard to look well, hoping to convey the thought that I'm not the type who seeks to magnify his illness.

Incredibly, some people have actually told me they were envious of my lifestyle. They wished they could do nothing but sleep and eat all day! It takes every ounce of self-control I can muster not to fall on my knees right there and ask the Lord to grant their request.

Other people send subtle signals of impatience. They say they are sympathetic, but their underlying message is "Why don't you try harder to beat this thing?" They don't understand that living with this illness is like being precariously balanced on a rickety old raft, swept up in the middle of an emotional and physical maelstrom. They don't see how hard I fight every day with all of my strength just to keep afloat. If these people really understood my illness, they would marvel at how strong I truly am. With insensitive people to deal with and bewildering situations to face, your loved one may begin to shy away from social situations. If you can run interference, helping people understand CFS and the way it affects your loved one, you will make social situations more enjoyable.

When people who are unfamiliar with CFS come to visit, it may be appropriate to take them aside and briefly explain the nature of the illness. Many people feel uncomfortable visiting people who are sick because they don't know what to say, or they may even feel guilty because they are well. You need to be the facilitator in awkward situations, trying to make everyone feel comfortable and at ease. In addition to explaining the illness to others, you can also make the needs of your loved one known. People are often nice enough to offer their help, but when a need arises, it is not always easy to ask. You can let people know how they can help, financially, physically, or emotionally.

## OFFERING YOUR HELP

It is very difficult to need financial help and even more difficult to receive it. If you want to help financially, you should consider having your loved one's bills delivered to you directly. This may alleviate some of the guilt involved and allow a greater sense of independence. Aside from helping your loved one financially, you may also want to make a contribution to one of the CFS organizations listed in Appendix D, or to one of the many facilities doing research on CFS.

Being active in the political arena is another way you can help. More funding is needed for CFS research, and public and government awareness needs to be raised. This means that a lot of letters need to be written to senators and representatives. My parents have taken over this chore for us. They have given hundreds of photocopied letters to friends, relatives, and associates to send to Washington. Many of our other relatives and friends have distributed letters in other states and districts. The various CFS organizations can provide you with names and addresses to write to.

## KEEPING UP TO DATE

When you are very ill, it is not easy to keep up on all the pertinent information on CFS. Our family and friends keep their eyes and ears open for any possible treatments or information that might help. They read articles and maintain correspondence with support groups and doctors.

Another way to show your support is by attending support group meetings with your loved one. It is wise for any family member or close friend to attend at least one meeting because it will help you understand the effects of CFS better. Since Shawn and I often feel too ill to attend meetings, my parents attend for us. This ensures that we don't miss any new information.

## SHARING THE BURDEN

Another important way to help your loved one is by helping with his or her physical needs. It is very difficult to ask for help from others because this illness persists for so many years. Maybe friends could alternate helping, one cooking a meal one week, another doing laundry, and so on. Coordinating all this help for your loved one is a valuable service, and perhaps you can even turn it into a social occasion if it isn't too draining.

## DON'T FORGET THE LITTLE THINGS

There are so many little but meaningful things you can do to encourage and support someone who is ill. In fact, your imagination is the only limitation to the ways you can lend your support. You could give flowers, CDs, books, bubble bath, favorite foods, cable TV, videos, or crafts. If your loved one is too ill to read, perhaps you could read a special book into a tape recorder.

Our friends and family know that our physical limitations make it very difficult to socialize. We find it draining to go out or to entertain. They overcome this by occasionally bringing a sub sandwich or a pizza, sharing a meal and some time with us.

Even a card or a phone call can give the encouragement needed to endure. When Shawn was too ill to leave the house or have anyone visit, mail was the highlight of her day. She desperately needed to know that other people cared. You can't imagine how intense this need is for people who are chronically ill. Some people who had never even met us sent us cards, letting us know they were praying for us. To know that someone cared enough to pray for us always touched us deeply. And please don't forget that touch is also an important way of expressing your love and concern, especially when your loved one is feeling isolated and alone.

## RECOGNIZING OTHER
## FAMILY MEMBERS' NEEDS

While it is important to do everything you can to be supportive of your loved one, it is just as important that you not neglect the other members of the family. Be sensitive to the way they are affected by this illness. They will be facing their own problems as well, and they should not be made to feel as if their struggles are unimportant. Their problems may not be as devastating as CFS is, but they are still painful and need to be acknowledged. And even though you are hurting for your loved one, it is important to allow other family members to be happy. They are growing and moving on; rejoice with them.

CFS is very demanding. While the syndrome is a constant, the symptoms and their severity seem to be in flux constantly. One day your loved one may be feeling better and the next he or she may be unable to perform the easiest of tasks. Each one of you must learn how to live with this devastating affliction. With everything you do and everything you say, try to imagine what it would be like to have CFS. If whatever you say or do is based in love, more than likely it will be received with gratitude and affection. My prayer for you is that, through this trial, your relationships will grow even closer.

* * *

I am sure that many of us with chronic fatigue syndrome wish we could sit down with a doctor who is truly knowledgeable about CFS and ask some questions, or find out about the latest treatments. However, most of us do not have access to CFS specialists in our area. The following three chapters, as well as the appendices, contain information from prominent CFS researchers who were kind enough to contribute to this book. It is a privilege to have them share their expertise with us.

# CHAPTER TEN

# Questions and Answers

Following is an interview with Anthony L. Komaroff, M.D., professor of medicine at Harvard Medical School and director of the Division of General Medicine and Primary Care, Department of Medicine at Brigham and Women's Hospital.

**Author:** Over the years, and throughout the world, chronic fatigue–like illnesses have been reported in medical literature. Do you think CFS is a new syndrome?

**Dr. Komaroff:** I believe that, most likely, CFS is an old syndrome that has different causes. Some of the causes could be new.

**Author:** Do you have any theories regarding the possible cause of CFS?

**Dr. Komaroff:** It is possible that CFS is triggered by chronic infections. I think many of the symptoms may be caused by subtle changes in brain chemistry and immune system chemicals. However, none of these theories is proven.

**Author:** Are there any diagnostic tests to help physicians when making a diagnosis?

**Dr. Komaroff:** Unfortunately, there are no very good diagnostic tests for CFS. There are a growing number of tests that produce abnormal results in many CFS patients, but no tests yet that are abnormal in all patients with this illness and normal in all individuals without it.

**Author:** You have always been a staunch supporter of the legitimacy of CFS. What have you seen in your patients that convinced you they were suffering from something other than depression?

**Dr. Komaroff:** Many patients with CFS simply do not meet the criteria for depression, nor do they get better with antidepressant therapy. Moreover, a number of objective biological measures are abnormal in many patients with CFS, but not in depression. Together, this evidence indicates to me that CFS is a biological or physical disorder that is different from depression.

**Author:** Over time, what percentage of your patients fully recover, and will the typical patient's symptoms tend to get better, worse, or stay the same?

**Dr. Komaroff:** In our experience, approximately ten to fifteen percent of patients have fully recovered from CFS. The vast majority of patients feel sickest in the first six to twelve months and improve to some degree over the course of time.

**Author:** Given the reports of CFS 'outbreaks,' such as reported in Lake Tahoe by Dr. Cheney, is chronic fatigue syndrome contagious?

**Dr. Komaroff:** There is no scientific proof that CFS is contagious. An outbreak that affects several people with the same kind of illness at about the same time does not necessarily mean an illness is contagious. For example, a toxin in the environment could do the same thing.

**Author:** The one question I am sure most anyone with CFS would want to ask you is which treatments have been most successful for your patients, and are there any particular ones you recommend?

**Dr. Komaroff:** Our experience with treatment has been greatest with low doses of tricyclic medications. In the very low doses we use, these medicines help improve the quality of sleep, and thereby improve some of the symptoms of CFS. Medications can also help control the pain that some patients experience with CFS.

**Author:** For anyone with a chronic illness, exercise is recommended by most physicians. And yet people with CFS tend to relapse with exercise. What kind of exercise regimen do you usually recommend?

**Dr. Komaroff:** I recommend that patients avoid becoming completely immobile; this leads to a deconditioned state that makes some of the symptoms worse. I recommend at least regular limbering or light aerobic exercises.

**Author:** Does rest tend to benefit patients?

**Dr. Komaroff:** Rest does tend to benefit patients, but complete inactivity is both physically and psychologically damaging.

**Author:** What is your advice to women with CFS who are considering pregnancy?

**Dr. Komaroff:** There is no evidence that pregnancy is harmful to a woman with CFS or her baby. Indeed, many women with CFS feel somewhat better during pregnancy. At the same time, raising a young child is exhausting for even the healthiest woman. A woman with CFS who is considering pregnancy should realize that the first several years after the baby is born will be particularly challenging for her.

**Author:** Is there any evidence of a family link or a genetic predisposition toward CFS?

**Dr. Komaroff:** There is no solid scientific evidence yet of a genetic predisposition.

**Author:** Is CFS linked to any other serious diseases, like cancer, arthritis, or AIDS?

**Dr. Komaroff:** There is no scientific evidence that CFS is linked to any other serious diseases.

**Author:** Do you think there is any connection between allergies and CFS, and can allergies make symptoms worse?

**Dr. Komaroff:** There appears to be a higher past history of allergies in patients with CFS, in most, but not all, studies.

**Author:** What is encephalitis, and how does it relate to CFS?

**Dr. Komaroff:** Encephalitis means inflammation of the brain. Strictly speaking, you can only diagnose encephalitis by examining brain tissue under a microscope, which is not indicated in CFS.

**Author:** In your opinion, how serious an illness is CFS?"

**Dr. Komaroff:** CFS interferes with a person's personal and work life. It is a serious illness.

**Author:** From a physician's viewpoint, what frustrates you most about CFS?

**Dr. Komaroff:** Any physician is frustrated when he or she does not have fundamental answers about an illness. This is true of CFS and, unfortunately, many other illnesses also.

**Author:** Can you briefly describe the findings of a possible link between CFS and hypotension?

**Dr. Komaroff:** There is evidence from research conducted at Johns Hopkins Medical School and by our own research group that some patients with CFS have abnormal control of blood pressure [leading to hypotension]. However, this is not true of all patients with CFS. We currently do not believe that successful treatment of such hypotension is a cure for CFS, although it may improve certain symptoms in some patients.

**Author:** Do you find that sleep disorders play a role in CFS, and is there anything patients can do to treat them?

**Dr. Komaroff:** Sleep disorders are quite common in CFS, and probably do contribute to the symptoms of the illness. Sleep disorders are of varying kinds requiring varying treatments. A patient's doctor, as well as doctors who are sleep specialists, can help with proper diagnosis and treatment.

**Author:** What do you see as the future of CFS; what can patients look forward to?

**Dr. Komaroff:** CFS clearly is a complex illness that probably does not have one single, simple cause. That means that progress will be difficult. Nevertheless, much progress has been made over the past ten years, and many more doctors and research scientists are now involved in studying CFS. I believe there will continue to be important progress in the coming years.

# CHAPTER ELEVEN

# A Doctor's Approach to Treating Chronic Fatigue Syndrome

BY

DAVID C. KLONOFF, M.D., F.A.C.P.
Clinical Professor of Medicine
University of California at San Francisco
San Francisco, California

Chronic fatigue syndrome is a real illness, and there are many effective treatments for it. My goal, as a doctor, is to mobilize my patients in order to expand the horizons of their lifestyle. I want to help my patients who are too ill to work get back to work. I want to help my patients who are working with the illness, but are too fatigued for anything except work and rest, to be able to enjoy their families, friends, and hobbies.

One of the concerns about chronic fatigue syndrome that I hear most often from my patients is that they heard chronic fatigue syndrome has no cure. Such a statement implies that nothing can be done to help patients who suffer from this syndrome. However, this is definitely not the case. My experience with chronic fatigue syndrome has been that a person's lifestyle often plays a part in the development of this illness and in the exacerbation of its symptoms. People who are leading an unhealthy lifestyle are at greater than average risk of developing chronic fatigue syndrome, or of making a slow recovery.

The illness is often triggered by an infection or by trauma. For example, one of my patients became ill after her car struck a wayward deer running across the freeway in the Silicon Valley of California.

Also, there is often a pattern of job stress, relationship problems, school problems, excessive time commitments, and too little attention to one's own needs at the onset of chronic fatigue syndrome. I refer to this group of folks as "twenty-five-hour-per-day people." After becoming ill, if these people continue to partake of these types of stressful activities excessively, or fail to slow down until they are comfortable with their lifestyles, then it will be very difficult to recover because stress generally exacerbates the multi-organ symptoms of chronic fatigue syndrome.

My reply to the question of whether there is a cure for this illness is that people who follow the recommended treatments and seek a less stressful lifestyle can significantly reduce the symptoms of chronic fatigue syndrome. It is a daily challenge to pursue a physically and emotionally healthy lifestyle. If former chronic fatigue syndrome patients do not care for themselves physically, or begin doing more than they can physically or psychologically handle, or if they fail to exercise, eat healthy foods, and allow enough time for sleep and for recreation, then they are at risk of a relapse. I believe chronic fatigue syndrome patients should not be seeking a cure, but rather control of their illness to achieve a happy, healthy life.

Many of my patients have been to see other physicians before me. Among the most common statements they report having heard are: (1) "There is nothing wrong with you"; (2) "The problem is in your head"; and (3) "You are depressed." The conclusion usually drawn from these statements is that the physician really means, "I think you are crazy." People with chronic fatigue syndrome are not crazy. The National Institutes of Health and the Centers for Disease Control and Prevention, as well as many medical centers across the country, are doing research on the nature of chronic fatigue syndrome, including its effects on the brain, hormone-producing glands, the immune system, and muscles. I have met very many dedicated scientists from NIH, CDC, and medical centers across the United States, as well as from foreign countries, who are working diligently to solve the mysteries related to chronic fatigue syndrome. These scientists would not be working on this illness unless they thought it was real. If you, the reader of this book, have chronic fatigue syndrome, once again, you are not crazy.

I divide treatment for chronic fatigue syndrome into two types: (1) nonpharmacologic, without the use of medications; and (2) pharmacologic, when medications are used. There is no reason to limit treatment to only nonpharmacologic or pharmacologic; both types are necessary. However, if I was only able to prescribe one or the other, I would choose the nonpharmacologic treatment. Remember, there is no known "magic bullet" cure for chronic fatigue syndrome. The treatment requires a little of this and of that.

## NONPHARMACOLOGIC TREATMENT

Nonpharmacologic treatment for chronic fatigue syndrome includes five areas: exercise, stress reduction, diet, a support group, and individual counseling.

1. Exercise is the most important treatment for chronic fatigue syndrome. My patients who suffer from this illness are almost always in a vicious downward cycle. They are fatigued with muscle pains and they have been getting a great deal of rest. A cycle develops whereby rest leads to muscle wasting, which leads to decreased performance, which leads to pessimism, which leads to disinterest in exercise, which in turn leads to even more rest. Daily exercise can end that downward cycle and replace it with an upward, positive cycle. When a person exercises, a new cycle develops consisting of exercise that leads to muscle enlargement, which leads to increased performance, which leads to optimism, which leads to interest in exer-

cise, which in turn leads to even more exercise. Studies have demonstrated that exercise has anti-anxiety and antidepressant properties. The reason may be a combination of producing endorphins (the pleasure hormone that our brains make when we exercise) and attaining a sense of accomplishment at having reversed the loss of function that befalls people with chronic fatigue syndrome. Of course, exercise is also beneficial for the cardiovascular system.

Exercise must be started slowly and increased gradually. If a person is generally fatigued and deconditioned, it is necessary to perform as much aerobic exercise as can be tolerated. Walking, swimming, riding a stationary bike, aerobic exercises from a videotape, or a rowing machine are all good aerobic exercises. I do not recommend weightlifting, which is anaerobic exercise. A person must exercise every day. Initially, the daily duration could be as little as five minutes, and even less in some cases. Each week the daily duration is increased by several minutes. After a few months, a person can be spending an hour or more per day exercising!

Avoid the pitfall of the overactivity-underactivity syndrome. This is what I call the tendency of a chronic fatigue syndrome patient to overdo it on days when he or she is feeling well, followed by an overall decline in performance. Inevitably, after unusually strenuous exercise, there will be severe pain and fatigue the next day, followed by several days of inability to do any exercise. The muscles will then waste away and the patient will have actually lost ground by the time he or she is ready to resume exercise. Studies have demonstrated an abnormal perception of muscular activity in chronic fatigue syndrome patients. They may not realize how much exercise they have done or when it is time to quit for the day. If a chronic fatigue syndrome patient is to regain muscle strength, it is necessary to perform a certain amount of exercise each day, recommended by his or her physician, and neither to underdo it nor overdo it.

2. Stress reduction is important to minimize the symptoms of chronic fatigue syndrome. Most of my patients report that stress makes their symptoms worse. Because there is no "magic bullet" cure, it becomes important to include any helpful activity in the treatment plan. Recognizing and avoiding stressful situations is important. An NIH panel recently advocated relaxation techniques and biofeedback for chronic pain (a condition that resembles chronic fatigue syndrome because lab tests and X rays are generally normal in both conditions, and yet patients may suffer greatly with both conditions). These treatments are also effective for chronic fatigue syndrome.

3. A well-balanced diet is part of the treatment for all chronic illnesses. Although chronic fatigue syndrome is not primarily a dietary disorder, like any debilitating illness it may lead to a disinterest in self-care and then to unhealthy dietary practices. Any patient interested in a very healthy diet can meet with a dietician or find books to read at the local library or bookstore. There are three points about diet for chronic fatigue syndrome that I, as an endocrinologist, feel strongly about. First, many patients with this syndrome also suffer from meal-induced hypoglycemia. They may feel weak, shaky, and sweaty a few hours after a meal. The symptoms tend to be provoked by large meals containing sweets and are relieved by eating. These hypoglycemic patients should avoid sweets and eat frequent small meals containing large amounts of starches and proteins, rather than one or two large meals each day. Second, many patients develop hypoglycemic symptoms from drinking caffeine. A study demonstrated that when a person drinks a diet soda with caffeine, compared to without caffeine, hypoglycemic symptoms will occur at higher blood-sugar levels. If the blood-sugar level in a patient is frequently on the borderline of being too low, then caffeine intake will render that person hypoglycemic. Thus, if you are prone to hypoglycemic symptoms, avoid caffeine. Third, there is no scientific validity to the concept that systemic candida or yeast is responsible for chronic fatigue syn-

drome, or that systemic candida even exists as an actual entity (except rarely in people with a serious disorder of the immune system). There is no reason to avoid foods containing yeast, sugar, or carbohydrates unless a patient cannot tolerate such a food because of a gastrointestinal disorder.

4. A support group can be very helpful for chronic fatigue syndrome patients. It must be led by a professional therapist, otherwise such a group may not be worth expending effort upon or may actually be harmful. In a support group, patients have a chance to deal with the stress of being affected by a chronic illness. Patients learn how to: (a) recognize and avoid situations that lead to exacerbation of symptoms; (b) seek help from other people; (c) relate better to their loved ones and understand the effects of the illness on their entire support system; and (d) attempt to enjoy life even while having this disabling condition. Patients will sometimes listen more closely to the comments of another patient rather than a physician because the other patient has "been in the same shoes" and can make suggestions about lifestyle based on personal experience.

5. Individual counseling allows any psychological issues that may accompany chronic fatigue syndrome to be explored in depth. Some patients are not comfortable speaking in front of a group. Others have so many issues to deal with that there is not enough time to discuss them in a group setting where everyone's concerns must be met. Also, some patients may have become extremely dysfunctional or depressed because of the illness and they may require intensive individual counseling, which is not available in a group. An ideal way for patients to improve their self-esteem and learn to lead a healthier lifestyle is to attend a support group as well as meet with a counselor on an individual basis. It is common for patients with chronic fatigue syndrome to have lost their job, their friends, their family ties, their financial stability, and in some cases their ability to concentrate, remember, or learn; at times, they may feel as if they are losing their minds. It is, therefore, not surprising to me

that many of these patients become depressed. It is not accurate to say that chronic fatigue syndrome is the same as depression, or that it is caused by depression; however, if depression is a symptom or consequence of the illness, then it should be treated.

## PHARMACOLOGIC TREATMENT

Pharmacologic treatment for chronic fatigue syndrome includes four areas: nonsteroidal anti-inflammatory drugs, symptomatic medications such as muscle relaxers and antispasmodics, tricyclic drugs, and selective serotonin re-uptake inhibitors (SSRIs). (Chronic fatigue syndrome patients are often sensitive to medications and may be prone to side effects unless low dosages are used in the beginning and the dosages can then gradually be increased.)

1. Nonsteroidal anti-inflammatory drugs are useful for the muscle and joint pains of chronic fatigue syndrome. Besides aspirin, it is now possible to purchase ibuprofen, naproxen, and ketoprofen over the counter. Many other anti-inflammatory drugs are more powerful and available by prescription only. These medications are often effective.

2. Symptomatic medication for treatment of muscle pains and spasms should include a muscle relaxer. Many of the muscle relaxers are sedating and best tolerated if taken after dinner or a few hours before bedtime so that any side effect of sleepiness will have worn off by the next morning. If a muscle relaxer is not sedating, then it can be used in the daytime as well. Many patients using a muscle relaxer would also benefit from daily stretching exercises to help overcome the inappropriate muscle spasticity that can occur. The muscles in the back of the neck and the bottom of the back of the skull (where the skull meets the back of the neck) frequently are tender and in spasm in chronic fatigue syndrome patients. With heat, muscle relaxers,

massage, vibration, stretching exercises, and in some cases home cervical traction, the headaches and stiff neck pains associated with this syndrome may be alleviated. Some patients suffer from an irritable bowel syndrome and benefit from antispasmodic medications as well as an increased amount of dietary fiber or a vegetable powder.

3. Insomnia frequently occurs in chronic fatigue syndrome. The tricyclic drugs, also known as tricyclic antidepressants, serve as effective, non-habit-forming sleeping pills. These medications shift the chemical balance of the brain and result in more sleep. They are effective for insomnia in low dosages, and for depression in low or high dosages. Just because an antidepressant is prescribed, it does not mean the physician is secretly diagnosing and treating depression, as well as ignoring a patient's physical complaints. Such a concern would be analogous to a situation whereby penicillin, which is used to treat syphillis and gonorrhea, would be labeled an anti–venereal disease drug and if a physician prescribed penicillin for a strep throat, the patient would question whether this means the physician is actually diagnosing venereal disease. If you are using a tricyclic drug such as amitriptyline, doxepin, desipramine, nortriptyline, or imipramine you should be aware of three potential side effects: (a) excessive sleep if the dose is too high, so start with a low dose and gradually increase the dose; (b) a dry mouth, so bring a glass of water to the bedroom at night; and (c) light-headedness upon rapid arising, so when arising at night to go to the bathroom or for any other reason, sit up slowly, then stand up slowly, then walk slowly, and hold on to furniture if necessary. Tricyclics not only help insomnia, which leads to fatigue, but are used by pain clinics to treat various states of chronic pain. They are also effective for fibromyalgia, which is a painful disorder of muscles and joints that is closely related to chronic fatigue syndrome.

4. A common symptom of this illness is hypersomnia, or excessive sleeping. A patient may sleep at night far more than

the adult average of approximately seven to eight hours nightly. Furthermore, such a patient may also require a daily nap. In a setting of excessive sleep, SSRI medications are very useful. These medications have been on the market in the United States for fewer than 10 years, but they have met a large need and are prescribed frequently. In 1995, 2 of the 10 most prescribed medications were SSRI medications, and these 2 medications alone accounted for 3 percent of total prescription revenue in the United States. These medications, in order of their age (oldest first), include fluoxetine, sertraline, paroxetine, and fluvoxamine. Venlafaxine is closely related to the SSRI medications. These medications are activating or stimulating. They are often effective. SSRI medications are also useful for patients who are obsessive/compulsive or overly concerned with details. Whereas most patients gain energy with these medications, a few patients complain of sleepiness and feel better with a bedtime dose rather than the typical morning dose. Even these patients report having more energy and needing fewer total hours of sleep. The SSRI medications have provided significant benefit to many patients with chronic fatigue syndrome.

There are many nonpharmacologic and pharmacologic treatments available for patients with chronic fatigue syndrome. Patients who use these treatments have the best outcomes. If a patient strives to treat the symptoms of chronic fatigue syndrome, and if a physician is truly ready to be sympathetic and help that patient, then it is possible over six to twelve months to make significant progress in overcoming this terrible, disabling illness.

# CHAPTER TWELVE

# Research Perspectives

BY
NELSON M. GANTZ, M.D., F.A.C.P.
Chairman of the Department of Medicine
and Chief of the Division of Infectious Diseases
Polyclinic Medical Center, Harrisburg, PA.
Clinical professor of medicine,
Pennsylvania State University
College of Medicine, Hershey, PA.

Since the first edition of this book was written, there has been an explosion in the research and papers published dealing with chronic fatigue syndrome. In 1988, a case definition of CFS was published. It was developed to provide a means of selecting patients to define this disorder better. Since its publication, there has been a revision of this definition, which was published in 1994. This new case definition was developed by investigators at the CDC and other researchers from all over the world. And, hopefully, it will permit researchers to better categorize patients with fatiguing illnesses to provide greater understanding of the causes and how to manage this difficult problem.

The etiology of CFS still remains unknown. Two reports published in 1987 suggested that Epstein-Barr virus was involved in causing this illness. However, reports published subsequently failed to show an important role for the Epstein-Barr virus in causing CFS. Similarly, a closely related virus, cytomegalovirus, is also not involved in causing CFS. Other etiologic agents such as human herpesvirus-6 and enteroviruses have also been suggested as etiologic agents. Human herpesvirus-6 appears to cause a childhood infection with fever and a skin rash called roseola, but it is unlikely to cause CFS. Several reports from England suggest an important role for enteroviruses such as Coxsackie virus as a cause of fatiguing illnesses. However, studies in this country have failed to establish that these viruses are causative agents of CFS. An initial report suggested that retroviruses were the cause of CFS, but again subsequent studies have failed to confirm this observation. Thus, at present, the etiology of CFS remains unknown. In addition to infectious agents, the syndrome may be precipitated by stress. Other investigators have focused on the importance of genetic influences as a cause of CFS, and research along this line is in progress.

In addition to pursuing infectious causes of CFS, other researchers have focused on endocrine abnormalities. In one study it appeared that adrenal gland function may be slightly diminished in patients with CFS compared with healthy controls. Based on this report, another study is looking at low-dose hydrocortisone therapy, a steroid hormone, compared with placebo to treat patients meeting the case definition of CFS.

Another avenue of research has focused on neurally mediated hypotension as a cause of CFS. It appears that some patients with this illness, when placed upright from a lying position, have a drop in their blood pressure. This decrease appears to be associated with a number of symptoms, such as fatigue and dizziness, which are commonly seen in patients with CFS. Some of the patients who have had an abnormal drop in blood pressure using a tilt table test have responded to methods to increase their blood pressure, such as with drugs and avoiding salt restriction. Again, further research along these lines is in progress. A number of investigators have attempted to understand the pathogenesis of CFS by measuring levels of cytokines, substances produced by the body cells in response to many stimuli. These cytokines, or cell hormones, of which CFS patients have been noted to have abnormal levels, may be responsible for some of the symptoms of this syndrome. However, although at present these abnormalities should not be used as a basis for a test to diagnose CFS, further research showing the importance of cytokines in the pathogenesis of CFS is underway.

While tremendous effort has been directed to trying to find the cause and understand the pathogenesis of CFS, there has also been research directed at treating this disorder. A number of studies have been conducted that treat patients with fibromyalgia, an illness similar to CFS. Studies have demonstrated that certain medicines are beneficial in improving sleep. For example, low-dose amitryptiline (Elavil) given at bedtime helps decrease pain and improve sleep in patients with fibromyalgia. In addition, another drug called cyclobenzaprine (Flexeril) given at bedtime also improves sleep and decreases pain. Besides these medicines that treat sleep and decrease pain, antidepressants appear to be beneficial in treating depression associated with CFS. Although CFS should not be equated with depression, many patients with this disorder have a secondary depression and respond to these medicines (again, controlled trials using antidepressants are needed).

In addition to pharmacologic approaches to treating CFS, other research has focused on using cognitive behavior therapy to diminish symptoms in patients. Cognitive behavior therapy (CBT) attempts to alter attitudes, perceptions, and beliefs that can contribute to maladaptive behavior. In a study of CFS patients treated by CBT and graded exercise, half experienced sustained improvement in functioning for six months. In a controlled trial, CBT, in combination with a graded exercise program, reduced symptoms and increased activity in patients with fibromyalgia as well.

CFS is a devastating illness for those who suffer from it. It is encouraging to see the explosion in the research focusing on the cause, the pathogenesis, and treatments of this disorder. Unfortunately, research is a slow process. Hopefully, further advances can be made to alleviate the suffering of those with this chronic waxing and waning illness.

# Epilogue

It is difficult to try to put the finishing touches on a book about my illness when my illness has no finish. This book is about my travail with CFS. The story can never truly have an ending until my illness has an ending.

I pray that this ending comes soon, for all of us. Until that time does come, we are forced to place some of the best parts of our lives on hold. In a sense, each one of us is waiting to live, longing to exhilarate in what most others take for granted: good health. For living and health go hand in hand.

Though some of our highest hopes and brightest dreams may be painfully beyond our grasp, we still must try to make the best of every day. Unfortunately, there is no easy way of making the best of CFS. In fact, the most difficult chapter to write in this entire book was the one on coping. I felt hypocritical, knowing that there are not enough chapters in all the books in all the libraries of the world to make coping with this affliction truly easy. The best I could hope to do was to bare a part of my soul so that you could see there is someone else who knows what you are going through—to try to encourage you by sharing some of the ways I have learned to cope with my illness. When all is said and done, however, you are the only one who can cope with your illness; no one can do it for you. Others can help make the burden a little lighter, but it's still your burden.

There is a wonderfully moving, anonymous poem entitled "Footprints in the Sand" about a man who dreams about his life. He sees two sets of footprints, one belonging to him and one belonging to God. He notices that during the lowest and saddest times in his life, there is only one set of footprints. Feeling betrayed and abandoned, he cries to God, "Lord, you said that once I decided to follow you, you'd walk with me all the way. But I have noticed that during the most troublesome times in my life, there is only one set of footprints. I don't understand why, when I needed you most, you would leave me." God replied, "My precious, precious child, I love you and I would never leave you. During those times of trial and suffering, when you saw only one set of footprints, it was then that I carried you."

Because of the faithfulness of God, the love of Shawn, and the support of family and friends, I have been carried through the trials of this illness more times than I can count. Till my dying day, I will never forget those who walked beside me, and for me, when I could not walk alone or at all.

Many images have been impressed upon my heart during the painfully long years of this affliction. The one that stands out most vividly, however, comes from the precious spirit of one sick little boy. I don't know his name and I met him only briefly, but the impact he has had on my life has been profound.

I met this boy during a hospital visit, when I used to go to New Jersey to take gamma globulin treatments. CFS patients were treated in the pediatrics wing of the hospital, and, as was usually the case, there were too many patients that day and too few rooms. While Shawn and I were in the waiting room, an adorable little boy walked up to me. He was around five years old, with big brown eyes and a disarming smile. I do not know what disease he was suffering from because neither he nor his mother spoke English. We did share a common language though: the language of the unwell.

He played make-believe doctor, and I was his patient. This little five-year-old was able to imitate hospital procedure flaw-lessly. In the world of imagination, he took my pulse, put a tourniquet around my upper arm, and performed a blood test. Next, he unwrapped a make-believe IV needle and inserted it in my arm, in the right place and in the right direction. Then he started a make-believe IV pump. After the "treatment" was complete, he reversed the procedure, removing everything in the proper sequence. Finally, with obvious gentleness and concern, he placed a make-believe Band-Aid at the site where the IV needle had been.

My eyes filled with tears then, and do so again even as I write. Here was a little boy so obviously acquainted with pain and suffering that hospital procedures were indelibly imprinted on his little heart—a heart tiny in size, but filled with immense love. As he left with his mother to see his doctor, I couldn't help but picture everything he had just done to me in his make-believe world—this time happening in painful reality. I could imagine his little bottom lip quivering, with tears welling in his big brown eyes, as doctors treated him for a disease he could not comprehend, with needles and medications he could only perceive as hurtful, not helpful. Yet, through everything he had obviously suffered, his eyes showed not the slightest hint of bitterness, resentment, or self-pity.

Whenever I start feeling sorry for myself, or bitter and resentful, I try to remember that little boy. For all of his short life he has known suffering, yet his spirit was as pure and gentle as any I have ever known. My highest aspiration is that my spirit may become as inspirational to others as that little boy's was to me. There is nothing about suffering that I don't loathe. But if I must suffer, I pray that it may make me a better person rather than a bitter one. My prayer for you is the same.

# Acknowledgments

A book is very rarely the product of one person. If this is true for healthy authors, it takes on a whole new meaning when the author is ill. This book has my name on it because it relates my struggle with CFS, but many people deserve to share the credit for writing it. I would especially like to thank Bernard and Mary Fisher and Caren Heacock for their assistance in writing, editing, rewriting, and typing the manuscript; Diana Baroni and Karen Thompson for their insightful editing of this edition; and Charles Conrad and Warner Books for believing in this book.

I am indebted to Drs. Oleske, Komaroff, Gantz, Klonoff, and Cheney, who were kind enough to contribute to this book. I want to thank Dr. Stephen Straus and Janet Dale, R.N., for their unwavering concern, not only for Shawn and me but for everyone who suffers with CFS.

I would also like to express my gratitude to some of the many people who have lovingly given their support over the long years of this illness. To my precious wife, Shawn, who makes each day better than the one before and means more to me than she will ever know. To my parents, Mary and Bernard, whose sensitivity and love see me through every day. To Caren and Eric, John Barlass, Lou Barlass, and Aunt Dory and Uncle Ralph, who are always there when we need them. To our special friends, Greg and Julie, Scotty and Lisa, Ken and Karen, Roy and Betty, Brenda and Greg, Rita and Sam, Pat and Eddie, Molly and Fred, Chris and Laura, and Alexander and Joel. To Mikaela, Joy, Charity, Jacob, Faith, David, Derek, Steven, Jenna, and Kevin, who have spent most of their lives praying for us. To Bob, Sybil, Janet, Judy, Rich and Dar, Orvalene, and our other CFS friends. Special thanks to Dr. Berman, Dr. Matook, Dr. Baker, Dr.

Deutsch, and Dr. Dahl. To everyone at the *Montclair Times*, Nancy, Sara, Donna, Jerry, Wood Graphics, and Phyllis. To Scott and Sharon, Dan and Barb, Darlene, the Voltmer cousins, the Olsens, Snappy, Bob, Laurie, Corpus, Community Christian Fellowship, and Mattituck Presbyterian Church. Thanks to all those who have been praying for us. Finally, I want to give all glory and honor to God, who makes life worth living no matter what the circumstances.

# APPENDIX A

# Gregg Fisher's Doctor Talks to Yours

What follows is an updated memo written by my doctor, James M. Oleske, for physicians of patients with chronic fatigue syndrome. If your physician hasn't had much experience with CFS, you might want to share this memo with him or her.

BY
JAMES M. OLESKE, M.D., M.P.H.
Francois-Xavier Bagnoud Professor of Pediatrics
Director, Division of Allergy, Immunology and
Infectious Diseases
Department of Pediatrics—UMD—New Jersey
Medical School

## BACKGROUND

Since 1980, several new or reemerging diseases have made an impact on the health of our communities and have challenged the responsiveness of the U.S. health-care system. The most obvious and lethal has been human immunodeficiency virus (HIV) infection, with its progression to the acquired immune deficiency syndrome (AIDS). Other emerging problems include

Lyme disease, penicillin-resistant pneumococcus infection, multiple-drug-resistant enterococcal infection, and the resurgence of tuberculosis (Tbc) and multiple-drug-resistant (MDR) forms of Tbc. Somewhat overshadowed, but still disabling both physically and psychologically, has been chronic fatigue syndrome (CFS), also known as chronic fatigue and immune dysfunction syndrome (CFIDS).

Patients with CFS have a confusing multi-organ system illness, the hallmark of which is disabling fatigue over long periods of time. Complicating this syndrome are a variety of other symptoms including poor concentration, memory loss, low-grade fever, headache, sleep disorder, muscular pain, and gastrointestinal upset.

In the past, there have been multiple descriptions of both endemic and epidemic outbreaks of prolonged fatigue illnesses: In 1750 one of the initial descriptions of a chronic fatigue illness was febricula ("little fever"), also known as vapors; by the 1800s, chronic fatigue was considered to be a weakness of the nerves—neuromyasthenia, also known as deCosta's syndrome. From the 1900s to the present, a number of syndromes and outbreaks of illnesses associated with chronic fatigue were described, including epidemic neuromyasthenia (Iceland disease, royal free disease, and others), postviral fatigue syndrome, chronic brucellosis, chronic mononucleosis-like syndrome, chronic Epstein-Barr virus (CEBV) infection, fibromyalgia syndrome, total allergy syndrome, tension fatigue syndrome, environmental allergy, and the "yeast connection."

As confusing as the individual symptoms of CFS are to the physician, so are the usual lack of collaborating physical findings and nondiagnostic laboratory studies. Frustration and secondary depression are frequent components to the patient who has already seen a number of general physicians as well as specialists. Many physician encounters with such patients are characterized by an all-too-brief history, curtailed physical exam, and limited laboratory evaluation. The diagnostic outcome is predictable: The patient's illness is diagnosed as depression, psychosomatic illness, or malingering.

Because of limited published studies of CFS, the evaluating physician has little available literature on which to base a specific diagnosis. Since 1988 there has been an increasing number of scientifically sound studies examining the epidemiology, natural history, and etiopathogenesis of CFS, which will help define the parameters of this syndrome. The *Annals of Internal Medicine* published an initial clinical case definition for CFS in May of 1988, which was revised in December 1994.

# 1988 CASE DEFINITION OF CHRONIC FATIGUE SYNDROME (CFS)

A case of chronic fatigue syndrome must fulfill both major criteria listed below, and the following minor criteria: 6 or more of the 11 symptom criteria and 2 or more of the 3 physical criteria; or 8 or more of the 11 symptom criteria.

## MAJOR CRITERIA

1. New onset of persistent or relapsing, debilitating fatigue, or easy fatigability in a person who has no history of similar symptoms, that does not resolve with bed rest, and that is sufficiently severe to reduce or impair average daily activity below 50 percent of the patient's activity before onset, for a period of at least 6 months.
2. Other clinical conditions that may produce similar symptoms must be excluded by thorough evaluation, based on history, physical examination, and appropriate laboratory findings. These conditions include malignancy, autoimmune disease, localized infection (such as endocarditis, Lyme disease, or tuberculosis), fungal disease (such as histoplasmosis, blastomycosis, or

coccidioidomycosis), and parasitic disease (such as toxoplasmosis, amebiasis, giardiasis, or helminthic infestation); disease related to HIV infection; chronic psychiatric disease, either newly diagnosed or by history (such as endogenous depression, hysterical personality disorder, anxiety neurosis, schizophrenia, or chronic use of major tranquilizers, lithium, or antidepressive medications); chronic inflammatory disease (such as sarcoidosis, Wegener's granulomatosis, or chronic hepatitis); neuromuscular disease (such as multiple sclerosis or myasthenia gravis); endocrine disease (such as hypothyroidism, Addison disease, Cushing syndrome, or diabetes mellitus); drug dependency or abuse (such as alcohol, controlled prescription drugs, or illicit drugs); side effects of a chronic medication or other toxic agent (such as a chemical solvent, pesticide, or heavy metal); or other known or defined chronic pulmonary, cardiac, gastrointestinal, hepatic, renal, or hematologic disease.

## MINOR CRITERIA

Symptom Criteria For inclusion in the definition of a case, a symptom must have begun at or after onset of fatigue, and must have persisted for at least 6 months (individual symptoms may or may not have occurred simultaneously):

1.  Mild fever (37.5°C to 38.6°C) or chills
2.  Sore throat
3.  Painful lymph nodes
4.  Unexplained generalized muscle weakness
5.  Muscle discomfort or myalgia
6.  Prolonged (24 hours or greater) generalized fatigue after levels of exercise that would have been easily tolerated before the onset of chronic fatigue

7. Generalized headaches (of a type, severity, or pattern that is different from headaches the patient may have had before onset of the chronic fatigue)
8. Migratory arthralgia without joint swelling or redness
9. Neuropsychologic complaints (one or more of the following): sensitivity to light, temporary visual blind or dark spots, forgetfulness, excessive irritability, confusion, difficulty thinking, inability to concentrate, depression
10. Sleep disturbance (hypersomnia or insomnia)
11. Description of main symptom complex as initially developing over a few hours to a few days (This is not a true symptom, but may be considered as equivalent to the above symptoms in meeting the requirements of the case definition.)

## PHYSICAL CRITERIA
1. Low-grade fever (oral temperature between 37.6°C and 38.6°C, or rectal temperature between 37.6°C and 38.6°C)
2. Nonexudative pharyngitis
3. Palpable or tender anterior or posterior cervical or axillary lymph nodes (Note: lymph nodes greater than 2 cm in diameter suggest other causes. Further evaluation is warranted.)

# 1994 REVISED CASE DEFINITION OF CHRONIC FATIGUE SYNDROME (CFS)

The revised case definition of the chronic fatigue syndrome is modeled on the 1988 chronic fatigue syndrome working case definition. The purpose of these revisions was to address some of the criticisms of that case definition and to facilitate a more systematic collection of data internationally. All physical signs were dropped from the inclusion criteria because it was agreed that their presence had been unreliably documented in past studies and the required number of symptoms was decreased from 8 to 4 and the list of symptoms was decreased from 11 to 8.

## MAJOR CRITERIA

A case of chronic fatigue syndrome must include the presence of the following:

1. Clinically evaluated, unexplained, persistent, or relapsing chronic fatigue that is of new or definite onset (has not been lifelong); is not the result of ongoing exertion; is not substantially alleviated by rest; and results in substantial reduction in previous levels of occupational, educational, social, or personal activities.

2. Other clinical conditions that may produce similar symptoms must be excluded by thorough evaluation, based on history, physical examination, and appropriate laboratory findings. These conditions include malignancy, autoimmune disease, localized infection (such as endocarditis, Lyme disease, or tuberculosis), fungal disease (such as histoplasmosis, blastomycosis, or coccidioidomycosis), and parasitic disease (such as toxoplasmosis, amebiasis, giardiasis, or helminthic infestation; disease related to HIV infection; chronic psychiatric disease, either newly diagnosed or by history (such as endogenous depression, hysterical personality disorder, anxiety neurosis, schizophrenia, or chronic use of major tranquilizers, lithium, or antidepressive medications); chronic inflammatory disease (such as sarcoidosis, Wegener's granulomatosis, or chronic hepatitis); neuromuscular disease (such as multiple sclerosis or myasthenia gravis); endocrine disease (such as hypothyroidism, Addison disease, Cushing syndrome, or diabetes mellitus); drug dependency or abuse (such as alcohol, controlled prescription drugs, or illicit drugs);

side effects of a chronic medication or other toxic agent (such as a chemical solvent, pesticide, or heavy metal); or other known or defined chronic pulmonary, cardiac, gastrointestinal, hepatic, renal, or hematologic disease.

## MINOR CRITERIA

Symptom Criteria The concurrent occurrence of four or more of the following symptoms, all of which must have persisted or recurred during 6 or more consecutive months of illness and must not have predated the fatigue:

1. Self-reported impairment in short-term memory or concentration severe enough to cause substantial reduction in previous levels of occupational, educational, social, or personal activities
2. Sore throat
3. Tender cervical or axillary lymph nodes
4. Muscle pain
5. Multijoint pain without joint swelling or redness
6. Headaches of a new type, pattern, or severity
7. Unrefreshing sleep
8. Post-exertional malaise lasting more than 24 hours

The method used to establish the presence of these and any other symptoms should be specified.

## PHYSICAL CRITERIA
None

# CFS AND ITS RELATIONSHIP TO IM ("MONO")

CFS may be caused by a number of different virus infections resulting in immune dysfunction and persistent inflammatory reactions that cause the complex and multiple symptoms of CFS. The human DNA herpesviruses, with their ability to maintain a latent lifelong infection with periods of reactivation, are strong candidates for being one of the causes of CFS. The similarities between the prolonged fatigue-like illness that can complicate acute infectious mononucleosis (IM) due to Epstein Barr virus (EBV) in the older child or adolescent and CFS, usually described in adults, led to the initial suspicion that EBV was a candidate as the etiological agent of CFS. The findings in early studies of CFS patients demonstrating a distinctive EBV serological response supported this assumption. Subsequent studies of larger numbers of patients with CFS, however, did not consistently demonstrate this unique serological response, while demonstrating that there may be other viral causes of CFS in addition to EBV.

In 20 percent of the patients I have evaluated for CFS, in addition to high EBV titers, I have seen concomitant increased cytomegalovirus (CMV) IgG titers. More recently even a greater percentage of CFS patients (80 percent) have serological evidence of past human herpesvirus-6 (HHV6) infection. It is possible that CFS may result from the interaction of more than one latent viral infection and subsequent abnormal immune responses. There have been additional studies linking CFS to disturbance in the neuroendocrine axis, with possible defects in ACTH- releasing factor and consequently an instability in cortisol levels.

## EVALUATING IM AND CFS PATIENTS

Based on a review of the literature and my own experience, I would urge the physician evaluating a patient with complaints of chronic fatigue to consider the following guidelines (Table 1): Allow enough time for an adequate history (at least $^1/_2$ hour) and prior to the initial patient visit, make every attempt to obtain any previous medical records. The initial encounters with the physi-

**TABLE 1**
**Evaluation of Patients Presenting with**
**Chronic Fatigue Syndrome**

Initial Evaluation

- Review previous medical records, reports and laboratory studies.
- Take a detailed history, including past history of other fatigue-like illness, significant psychiatric illness, detailed review of symptoms (see Table 3, page 199) and determine what pattern of illness patient has been experiencing (see Figure 1, A & B).
- Perform a thorough physical exam.
- Laboratory studies: CBC with sed rate, SMA18, thyroid functions, ANA, UA, EKG, chest X ray and intermediate strength PPD. If fever is over 101°, obtain several blood cultures.
- Other studies: CAT or MRI brain scan, psychological testing

Further Evaluations

- Follow-up of any abnormalities found on initial workup to define other causes of chronic fatigue (Table 2)
- Appropriate subspecialist referral after initial evaluation
- Research/ID-immunology evaluation to include: serological evaluation for infectious agents, CMV, EBV, HHV6, and others (Table 2), humoral immune evaluations (IgG, M, A, and E levels, IgG subclass levels), and cellular immune evaluations (T-cell subsets evaluation)

* Regular repetition of most laboratory studies is usually not appropriate.

cian for the patient with CFS should be devoted to differential diagnosis to ensure that the suspected CFS patient's multiple complaints are not due to other causes (see Table 2). This workup of exclusion needs to include selected laboratory studies guided by a thorough history and careful physical exam.

## CLINICAL EVALUATIONS: PATTERNS OF IM AND CFS

Since 1976, I have had experience in evaluating over 200 older children, adolescents, and adults presenting with significant and chronic fatigue-like illnesses and would offer the following observations that may be helpful in recognizing the clinical presentations that characterize patients with CFS as well as

---

**TABLE 2**

**The Differential Diagnosis in Patients Presenting with CFS**

- Persistent infectious mononucleosis
- Autoimmune diseases such as fibromyalgia/other collagen-vascular diseases, including Behçet's and Sjögren's syndromes
- Neuromuscular disease, including multiple sclerosis and myasthenia gravis
- Chronic inflammatory diseases, including Chron's disease, sarcoidoisis and Wegener's granulomatosis
- Chronic infections such as Lyme disease, hepatitis A/B/C, HIV infection, chronic brucellos, subacute bacteria endocarditis, tuberculosis
- Fungal/parasitic diseases
- Chronic asthma/allergic illnesses
- Adult-onset cystic fibrosis
- Chronic psychiatric illness
- Endocrine disease
- Drug dependency
- Environmental toxins
- Lymphoma and other hidden malignancies
- Sleep apnea

---

older children and adolescents with prolonged or recurrent EBV-associated IM:

There are several similarities between adults (usually over 24 years of age) meeting the diagnostic criteria of CFS and young adults, adolescents, and older children diagnosed with IM. Both are illnesses that cause significant fatigue, can persist for longer than 6 months, and can be associated with other symptoms. Figure 1 depicts the various patterns of fatigue seen in both IM (Figure 1-A) and CFS (Figure 1-B). Patients with acute IM present with one or more signs and symptoms, including exudative tonsilitis, enlarged lymph glands, hepatosplenomegaly, encephalitis, carditis, dermatitis, hemolytic anemia, thrombocytopenia, jaundice, fever, and fatigue. This acute viral

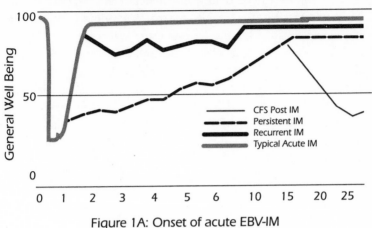

Figure 1A: Onset of acute EBV-IM

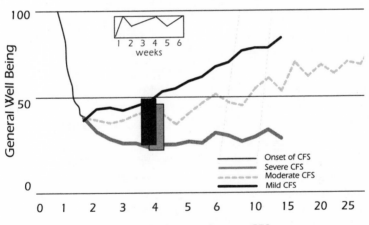

Figure 1B: Onset of acute CFS

infection with EBV is well characterized (Pattern A-1, Typical Acute IM), but there remains a general lack of appreciation as to how severe and prolonged a bout of acute EBV mononucleosis may be for an individual patient. I have seen several adolescent patients who have experienced periodic flare-ups of sore throat, cervical adenopathy, and fatigue 2 to 4 years after the initial bout of acute IM (Pattern A-2, Recurrent IM). Some patients may have persistence of symptoms, especially fatigue, for 3 to 5 years after a severe bout of acute EBV infection (Pattern A-3, Persistent IM). In general, however, such adolescent and young adult patients completely recover and do not progress to what has been called CFS or CFIDS. Only a longer period of observation of such patients will answer the question of the relationship among the severity of acute IM, treatments given, and the development of CFS later in life (Pattern A-4, CFS post-IM?).

CFS usually occurs in young adults, and in females more frequently than males. In our initial group of 80 patients meeting the 1988 diagnostic criteria for CFS, the mean age was 28 years with a range of 12 to 50 years. There was a female-to-male ratio of cases of 2:1. Table 3 lists the signs and symptoms we have seen in our group of CFS patients.

Frequently patients with CFS give a history of acute IM, but usually several years in the past, with an intervening history of good health. The onset of CFS usually begins as a flulike illness from which the patient never completely recovers. The major symptoms appear related to CNS dysfunction, a flulike illness with arthralgia and GI upset. A general pattern that I have seen is an initial arthralgia flulike illness that becomes progressively worse with fatigue and other symptoms, which peak in severity at 1 to 3 years. Thereafter, there may be a gradual improvement in symptoms over the next 5 to 10 years (Pattern B-1, Mild CFS). This pattern is similar to that seen in persistent IM (Pattern A-3, Persistent IM). The true course of recovery varies greatly from patient to patient. There is frequent exacerbation of symptoms, during which patients feel they are again as sick as before. However, when patients evaluate their symptoms more objectively, it is recognized that there has been a slow but gradual recovery from CFS over several years. Some individuals never fully recover to full function. Other patients have greater fluctuation in symptoms over the course of their CFS (see Figure 1B insert) with

### TABLE 3
#### Clinical Signs and Symptoms in 80 CFS Patients

| | |
|---|---|
| Fatigability | (80)—100% |
| Depression | (73)—90% |
| Body Weakness | (70)—87% |
| Headache | (57)—71% |
| Decreased Concentration/Memory | (52)—65% |
| Glandular Swelling (L.N.) | (52)—65% |
| School/Job Failure | (50)—63% |
| Fever | (42)—52% |
| Sore Throat | (42)—52% |
| Abdominal Pain/Cramps | (34)—43% |
| Arthralgia/Stiff Joints | (33)—41% |
| Allergy-like Symptoms | (28)—35% |
| Body Aches/Myalgia | (28)—35% |
| Confusion | (21)—26% |
| Lethargy | (21)—26% |
| Rash | (14)—17% |
| Puffy Eyelids | (14)—17% |
| Nausea | (14)—17% |
| Hepatosplenomegaly | (14)—17% |
| Blurring Vision/Photophobia | (10)—13% |
| Dizziness | (10)—13% |
| Swelling Hands | (9)—11% |
| Diarrhea | (7)—9% |
| Shortness of Breath | (7)—9% |
| Suicidal Attempt | (3)—4% |
| Clumsiness | (3)—4% |
| Hair Loss | (3)—4% |
| Hallucination | (3)—4% |
| Raynaud's Phenomenon | (2)—2% |
| Recurrent Aseptic Meningitis | (2)—2% |
| Slurred Speech | (2)—2% |
| Tinnitus | (2)—2% |
| Loss of Taste and Smell | (2)—2% |

# TREATMENT INFORMATION

## Medications, Herbal Preparations, and Miscellaneous Treatments That Have Been Used Against Chronic Fatigue Syndrome

(SOURCE: CDC "FACTS ABOUT CFS")

### Vitamins, Co-enzymes and Minerals

| Treatment Name | Value in Treating CFS* | Side Effects Associated with the Use of This Treatment |
|---|---|---|
| Co-enzyme Q-10 | F | Harmful effects unknown |
| Vitamin B-12 | X | Harmful effects unknown |
| Vitamin C | X | Long-term use of high dose may cause development of kidney stones. |
| Vitamin A | X | High doses of this vitamin may cause a wide variety of clinical symptoms, including permanent liver damage. |
| Selenium | X | Compounds of this element may cause gastrointestinal disturbances, and some are carcinogenic. |
| Germanium | X | Harmful effects unknown |
| Zinc | X | Harmful effects unknown |
| Iron | X | High doses of iron salts may be toxic. |
| Adenosine monophosphate | F | Harmful effects unknown |
| Magnesium | X | Harmful effects unknown |
| L-tryptophan | F | Contaminated lots have been implicated in triggering eosinophilia-myalgia syndrome. |

*X = No proven utility for CFS; F = No known clinical value

### Herbal Preparations

| Treatment Name | Value in Treating CFS* | Side Effects Associated with the Use of This Treatment |
|---|---|---|
| Astragalus | X | Harmful effects unknown |
| Echinacea | X | Harmful effects unknown |
| Garlic | X | Harmful effects unknown |
| Ginseng | X | Moderate use considered safe, but allergic reactions have been reported. High doses may cause a variety of adverse symptoms. |

## Herbal Preparations (continued)

| Treatment Name | Value in Treating CFS* | Side Effects Associated with the Use of This Treatment |
|---|---|---|
| Ginkgo biloba | F | Harmful effects unknown |
| Comfrey | X | Contains tannin and lasiocarpine, both of which are considered carcinogenic. Alkaloids in comfrey may result in liver damage. |
| Primrose oil | C | Harmful effects unknown |
| Shiitake mushroom extract | F | Harmful effects unknown |
| Borage seed oil | F | Harmful effects unknown |
| Quercetin | X | Harmful effects unknown |
| Bromelain | X | "Therapeutic doses" may cause nausea, vomiting, diarrhea, skin rash and menorrhagia. |

*X = No proven utility for CFS; F = No known clinical value; C = Conflicting findings in clinical trials

## Analgesics

| Treatment Name | Value in Treating CFS* | Examples | Side Effects Associated with the Use of This Treatment |
|---|---|---|---|
| Nonsteroidal anti-inflammatory drug (NSAID) | S | Naproxen Ibuprofen Piroxicam | Abdominal pain, dyspepsia, nausea/vomiting, drowsiness, headache, depression, fatigue. Naproxen may impair some immune functions. |
| Other | S | Cyclobenzaprine | Gastrointestinal bleeding, drowsiness, dry mouth, dizziness |

*S = Useful for relief of symptoms

## Acute Analytics

| Treatment Name | Value in Treating CFS* | Examples | Side Effects Associated with the Use of This Treatment |
|---|---|---|---|
| Benzodiazepines | S | Alpraxolam Lorazepam | Sedation, anterograde amnesia, withdrawal symptoms |
| Other | S | Buspirone | Dizziness, headache, drowsiness, nausea |

*S = Useful for relief of symptoms

## Hypnotics

| Treatment Name | Value in Treating CFS* | Examples | Side Effects Associated with the Use of This Treatment |
|---|---|---|---|
| Benzodiazepines | S | Clonazepam Triazolam Temazepam | Hallucinations, ataxia, depression |
| Other | S | Zolpidem | Dizziness, headache |
| Other | S | Trazodone | Drowsiness, headache, gastrointestinal bleeding |

*S = Useful for relief of symptoms

## Antidepressants

| Treatment Name | Value in Treating CFS* | Examples | Side Effects Associated with the Use of This Treatment |
|---|---|---|---|
| Tricyclic antidepressants | S | Doxepin Amitriptyline Desipramine Nortriptyline | Dry mouth, drowsiness, weight gain, tachycardia, weakness, fatigue |
| Serotonin re-uptake inhibitors | S | Fluoxetine Sertraline Paroxetine | Headache, tremor, agitation, nervousness |
| Other | S | Bupropion | Anxiety, agitation, insomnia, tremor, anorexia, seizures |

*S = Useful for relief of symptoms

## Additional Drug Therapies

| Treatment Name | Value in Treating CFS* | Examples | Side Effects Associated with the Use of This Treatment |
|---|---|---|---|
| Calcium channel blockers | X | Nimodipine Nicardipine | Dizziness, hypotension, headache, nausea |
| H-2 blockers | X | Ranitidine Cimetidine | Headache, dizziness, nausea, rashes, myalgia, impotence, changes in immune function |
| Immune suppressants | U | Cyclophosphamide Azathioprine Methotrexate | Destruction of immune cells, hair loss, liver damage, kidney damage, toxicity to embryos, interstitial pneumonitis |
| Other | X | Naltrexone | Insomnia, liver damage |
| Other | X | Pentoxifylline | Gastrointestinal upset, dizziness |

*X = No proven utility for CFS; U = Use unjustified for CFS

## Allergy Medications

| Treatment Name | Value in Treating CFS* | Examples | Side Effects Associated with the Use of This Treatment |
|---|---|---|---|
| Nonsedating Antihistamines | S | Terfenadine Astemizole Loratadine | Drowsiness, interaction with erythromycin |
| Antihistamines | S | Diphenhydramine | Drowsiness |
| Other | S | Hydroxyzine | Sedation |

*S = Useful for relief of symptoms

## Miscellaneous Therapies

| Treatment Name | Value in Treating CFS* | Side Effects Associated with the Use of This Treatment |
|---|---|---|
| Gamma globulin | C | Harmful effects unknown |
| Ampligen | C | Harmful effects unknown |
| Kutapressin | X | Allergic reactions |
| Hydrogen peroxide injection | F | Stroke |
| High colonic enemas | F | Intestinal disease |

*X = No proven utility for CFS; F = No known clinical value; C = Conflicting findings in clinical trials

## Generic and Trade Names of Drugs Used to Treat Patients with CFS

| Generic Name | Trade Name |
|---|---|
| Alprazolam | Xanax |
| Amitriptyline | Elavil, Endep, Etrafon, Limbitrol, Triavil |
| Bupropion | Wellbutrin |
| Buspirone | BuSpar |
| Cimetidine | Tagamet |
| Clonazepam | Klonopin |
| Cyclobenzaprine | Flexeril |
| Desipramine | Norpramin |
| Doxepin | Adapin, Sinequan |
| Fluoxetine | Prozac |
| Lorazepam | Ativan |
| Nortriptyline | Aventyl, Pamelor |
| Paroxetine | Paxil |
| Pentoxifylline | Trental |
| Ranitidine | Zantac |
| Sertraline | Zoloft |
| Temazepam | Restoril |
| Trazodone | Desyrel |
| Triazolam | Halcion |
| Zolpidem | Ambien |

episodes lasting from 1 to 6 weeks, interspersed with periods of improvement, but never return to prior health status (Pattern B-2, Moderate CFS). During a flare-up of symptoms, such patients are usually so fatigued they can perform no useful tasks. Some patients may have continuous symptoms that are made worse by intercurrent illnesses or emotional or physical stress, and are unable to perform daily activities of living (Pattern B-3, Severe CFS).

I have not seen, nor has the medical literature reported, an increased incidence of malignancy or other life-limiting complications in patients with CFS. I have cared for eight women with CFS who became pregnant and had uneventful pregnancies with delivery of normal newborns. Six out of the eight women reported improvement in their CFS during pregnancy, and none of them showed worsening of their CFS postpartum.


## LABORATORY EVALUATIONS

At the very least, patients with suspected CFS should have a CBC differential and platelet count, sed rate, multiple blood chemistry, TSH, ANA, U/A, EKG, and chest X ray. If there are episodes of fever, patients should also have several blood cultures taken. A more aggressive FUO evaluation will need to be considered in patients with persistent episodes of fever. Patients with predominant CNS symptomatology suggesting a chronic encephalopathy (confusion, episodes of lack of concentration, headache, depression, and insomnia) may benefit from a more detailed neurological evaluation by a consultant neurologist that may include a CAT or MRI scan of the brain. Examination of spinal fluid is usually reserved for CFS patients suspected to have multiple sclerosis. It has recently been recommended that a more formal mental status examination be included as part of the workup for CFS as well as including both subjective and performance aspects of fatigue level and overall functional performance. Some of these instruments may not be appropriate for young adolescents and children, and physicians may need to collaborate with a clinical psychologist. Due to the chronicity of CFS, periodic measurement of quality of life should also be part of the overall evaluation.

A more intensive laboratory evaluation that would be performed as part of a research protocol or consultation by an infectious disease/immunology specialist on selected patients may include: assays for HHV6, CMV (IgM and IgG antibodies), EBV titers that examine for VCA-IgG and IgM antibodies, early antigen (restricted and diffuse) and EBNA titers. Based on my experience with humoral immune deficiency in patients with CFS, I also would recommend that selected patients with unexplained fatigue over 6 months of age have quantitative immunoglobulin (IgG,A,M,E) and IgG subclass levels performed. In 40 percent of the cases I have evaluated for CFS, there have been demonstrated depressed levels of total and subclass IgG levels. If these humoral immune studies are abnormal, such patients should be referred for further immune system evaluation.

While not part of the initial evaluation of patients with CFS, selected patients or participants in natural history studies may have cellular immune evaluations that include quantitative and qualitative analysis of lymphocyte subsets looking for patterns of both immune activation and immune suppression. Such abnormal patterns may show an increase in activation markers (CD38 and HLA-DR) on CD8+ cells with a reduction of the CD11B marker for suppressive cell activity. Recently a reduction in the percentage of naive CD4+ cells has been noted in CFS as well as a reduction in functional activity of natural killer (NK) cells. Though nonspecific, these latter studies have demonstrated a pattern that supports cellular immune dysregulation associated with CFS.

After the initial laboratory evaluations of the patient with suspected CFS is completed, there is little benefit in the routine repetition of viral serological assays.

## TREATMENT FOR CFS

There is no specific therapy for CFS. Antiviral trials with acyclovir have not demonstrated efficacy and have the potential to cause harm (e.g., renal disease). Symptomatic care and emotional support are important in improving the quality of life and general well-being of an individual with CFS. The best individual to coordinate this program would be a nonjudgmental and committed primary-care physician. CFS patients usually do poorly when they receive fragmented care from a number of subspecialists. Any patient with a chronic illness needs emotional support to manage the stress of their illness. Many patients with CFS would benefit from the techniques available through a psychologist (i.e., stress management, self-hypnosis, behavior modification, etc.). Only infrequently do such patients require referral to a psychiatrist.

As with any chronic illness, good nutrition is important, but CFS is not caused by a specific vitamin/mineral deficiency. A daily vitamin/mineral supplement is a reasonable recommendation, but high doses of intravenously administered vitamins is not recommended. Patients do benefit from limited exercise (therapeutic strengthening/breathing exercise, yoga) that gives a psychological lift but not so strenuous that it results in a relapse of more severe fatigue. Patients with CFS seem to have a greater risk of having exacerbation or onset of typical allergic diseases with onset of their CFS. Individuals experiencing the onset or worsening of asthma, rhinitis, conjunctivitis, and other inhalant allergic symptoms should receive appropriate allergic care, which may include the use of nonsedation antihistamines. Such antihistamines do not cross the blood-brain barrier and therefore do not exacerbate the fatigue as is the tendency of other classes of antihistamines. Additional allergic-based therapies and evaluations may be helpful, depending on the individual's specific symptoms. Many of the patients I have seen with CFS have insomnia or poor sleep habits despite feeling exhausted. Such patients may benefit from taking a tricyclic antidepressant before bedtime. I have used Doxepin, 10 to 75 milligrams, at night for many CFS patients, and over half felt marked improvement in sleep disturbance. Appropriate care, however, must be exercised in the use of these medications.

When headache is a major manifestation of a CFS patient, I have prescribed acetazolamide (Diamox sequels, 500 milligrams) taken 20 minutes prior to bedtime. This mild diuretic possibly lowers CFS pressure as it does in decreasing anterior eye chamber pressure in glaucoma and in preventing the symptoms of high-altitude exposure. Some patients complain of "tingling" in their hands with this drug, and it should not be used if there is a history of kidney stones. Patients treated with acetazolamide usually improve after a 2-week daily course and can be maintained on 2 to 3 doses a week with no significant side effects and continued improvement in headache symptoms.

The joint symptoms and generalized aches and pains that many patients with CFS experience will frequently be improved with a nonsteroidal anti-inflammatory agent. The use of steroids in CFS is controversial, and the serious side effects and toxicity of this hormone must always be considered. Only infrequently would the risks of using steroids be outweighed by possible benefits in a specific patient. The long-term risk of using steroids is a major therapeutic decision requiring careful evaluation of benefit and risk. For the patient with a chronic illness, such as CFS, the use of steroids has significant theoretical risks and little proven benefit. While considering the above, there have been rare circumstances when I have given a short course of prednisone to a patient with severe exhibition of CFS. The use of steroids in such cases may provide a short period of relief of symptoms, but the long-term use of prednisone even in a low-dose, alternate-day schedule is not to be recommended. In addition to prednisone, ACTH, and the cortisol metabolic intermediate dehydroepiandrosterone (DHEA), have been suggested as possible therapies for CFS. I have personal experience with 3 CFS patients who improved with long-term DHEA therapy (100 to 800 milligrams a day), but several other CFS patients showed no improvement after taking a course of DHEA.

When a patient with CFS is identified to have dysgammaglobulinemia, replacement therapy with intravenous gamma globulin (IVIG) needs to be considered. Approximately 40 percent of the patients I have seen with CFS demonstrate IgG or IgG subclass deficiency (usually IgG3). This group of patients, when treated with monthly IVIG (400 milligrams/kilograms/per dose), have had symptomatic improvement, usually beginning after the third dose, with less fatigue, sore throats, and cervical adenopathy. These patients may have some worsening of CFS symptoms during the first 3 months of IVIG therapy. I have treated patients who have responded positively to IVIG therapy for up to 3 years. The cost of IVIG is significant, and this limits its use to those patients with defined antibody deficiency associated with their CFS. When there are additional abnormalities found in cellular immune functions, such patients may be more appropriately classified as having common variable immunodeficiency syndrome. This immune deficiency diagnosis/classification is more likely to be accepted by health insurance and disability programs.

Patients with CFS may benefit by referral to nationally recognized CFS research centers. As the etiopathogenesis is defined by these research efforts, improved diagnostic laboratory assays will be developed. The lack of a specific etiology, however, should not preclude the development and performance of clinical treatment trials. Specifically, tricyclic antidepressants, acetazolamide, IVIG, anti-inflammatory agents, DHEA, and other modalities should be evaluated in controlled studies. The list of treatments on page 200 compiled by the Centers for Disease Control and Prevention should be evaluated by clinical research trials. Pending the performance of such clinical trials, it is appropriate for the primary-care provider to maintain an ongoing dialogue with the CFS patient regarding both patient- and physician-initiated therapy with various treatments, both traditional and nontraditional, as outlined in the CDC list of treatments (page 200).

## ROLE OF PRIMARY-CARE PROVIDERS IN THE CARE OF CFS PATIENTS

One role the physician caring for a patient with suspected CFS must include is advocacy. While recognizing that the physician must evaluate and suspect emotional/psychological illness and make appropriate referrals, many patients with CFS are suffering from a poorly understood organic syndrome probably related to chronic immune dysfunction initiated by a past, latent, or reactivated viral infection. Many of such patients' emotional distresses and depressions are reactive and related to their chronic organic illnesses and the frequent disbelief and frustration of physicians, friends, and family. It is the role of a primary-care physician to evaluate, offer supportive care that is appropriate, and help their CFS patient avoid victimization by "health" providers offering often expensive but unproven therapies. Constant referral to multiple specialists is usually not helpful to the patient or the primary-care doctor, especially if a careful preliminary evaluation is not initially performed. There are appropriate subspecialties that may be helpful in evaluation of the patient with chronic fatigue, including neurology, psychology, gastroenterology, rheumatology, rehabilitation, allergy/immunology, and infectious diseases. In patients under eighteen years of age, pediatric-trained subspecialists are preferable.

There are specific syndromes that are often confused with CFS in which such referrals are especially appropriate, such as fibromyalgia rheumatica, which should be diagnosed and managed in collaboration with a rheumatologist. In selected areas of the United States, Lyme disease is frequently diagnosed as the cause of chronic fatigue, especially when associated with arthralgia-like symptoms, despite the lack of any confirmatory laboratory studies. Without the help of an experienced infectious disease specialist, such patients misdiagnosed with Lyme disease are frequently given prolonged courses of unnecessary antibiotics before diagnosis of CFS is made.

## CONCLUSION

The primary-care physician should help a patient with CFS negotiate the difficult problems they will encounter with entitlement programs and managed-care organizations. Those patients who are disabled and unable to work need to have their physician provide supported documentation to the Social Security Administration. It is inappropriate for physicians to claim they "don't believe" that there is a chronic fatigue syndrome. Rather, patients presenting with prolonged fatigue require a careful and thorough evaluation. Whether the patient with disabling chronic fatigue symptoms suffers from an as yet poorly understood postviral systemic illness associated with reactive depression (somatopsychic) or a primary emotional illness (psychosomatic), they deserve to have a physician who will provide compassionate care and appropriate advice and referral while maintaining patient contact and advocacy.

# Appendix B

# CFS Research: Questions, Challenges, and Obstacles

BY

PAUL R. CHENEY, M.D., PH.D.,
The Cheney Clinic, Charlotte, North Carolina

Chronic fatigue syndrome (CFS) relates to a chronic, relapsing, and often evolving illness usually characterized by dysfunctional fatigue, recurrent pharyngitis, adenopathy, headache, low-grade fever, muscle and joint aches, cognitive disorders, and neuropsychiatric problems. Chronic fatigue and immunodysfunction syndrome (CFIDS) relates to that subcategory of CFS patients for whom objective evidence exists of significant immune dysfunction or perturbation. Whether these "abnormal findings" represent a primary immunologic defect resulting in loss of control of certain ubiquitous but usually latent viral infections, or are secondary to chronic active infection by an immunotropic virus, or are secondary to some other process cannot at present be determined with confidence. It is highly likely that these situations can exist separately, but vicious cycles may be set up that make it difficult to determine the exact causal agent or mechanism. The almost inevitable influence of cofactors, both endogenous (i.e., genetic or developmental) and exogenous (i.e., environmental or coinfections), makes this one of the most challenging disorders ever studied. Threads of new insight weave their way from CFS into a host of other medical conditions, both well defined and poorly defined. To study this disorder is in a sense to study a much larger part of medicine because many of the same elements can be seen in other diseases due to common physiologic and pathophysiologic pathways. However, the fact that CFS has erupted onto the medical landscape as a reasonably common, clinically recognizable condition that may also be on the rise raises an important question: Is there some new agent or factor driving most cases of CFS/CFIDS that have developed in the last ten or fifteen years?

Because of the usually abrupt-onset and mono-like clinical character as well as the serologic findings of increased Epstein-Barr virus (EBV) replication activity, this illness quickly assumed in the United States the label chronic Epstein-Barr virus syndrome (CEBV) or chronic mononucleosis syndrome. In a substantial number of patients, however, evidence of abnormal EBV activity is lacking, and a few patients with this syndrome are sero-negative for EBV. Despite lack of EBV ubiquity, which challenged its role as a cause of the syndrome, the Epstein-Barr virus will likely always be associated with this syndrome either as a secondary effect in most cases or as a primary cause of disease in an important but undetermined minority of CFS patients.

Recently, there has been a growing impression that CFS is increasing in frequency in the population. The syndrome may be well represented in the 20 percent of primary-care patients who complain of significant and prolonged fatigue of abrupt onset. Half of all patients given the diagnosis of fibromyalgia may find the label CFS a better fit. Outbreaks of this syndrome have been reported and strongly suggest that a novel agent or set of factors is at play in a virgin population. Indeed, the best candidate as a novel cause of CFS is the newly discovered human herpesvirus 6 or HHV6. The apparent laboratory behavior of HHV6 could, if present in this condition, allow it to eclipse EBV as an associated if not causal factor in CFS. There may well be other undiscovered infectious agents and cofactors that could combine to make this a true "witches' brew" of a problem. It is even possible that no single infectious agent or group of infectious agents is primarily responsible but that these agents are secondary effects of an environmental immunotoxin.

Beyond infectious agents and toxins lies the concept of stress. While stress can play a role in any disease, it may play a far more central role in CFS. Stress can clearly modulate the cycles of symptoms, promote relapse of symptoms, and is often implicated at the onset of this syndrome. The relationship of stress to CFS is clear enough to suggest it as a cofactor but probably not the cause of CFS. Too many patients have little or no stress involved at the onset or relapse of their symptoms.

Despite the increasing weight of evidence that this syndrome is a real disease with measurable immunologic, serologic, and neurologic abnormalities, many institutions and prominent physicians scoff at this problem and the patients who have it. It is therefore important to move quickly to establish ever more objective markers for this syndrome and to search out its basic pathophysiology and ideally its cause(s). Quite apart from the professional divisions over this syndrome, this could be a very serious and widespread health problem.

Probably the most important question about CFS is whether or not its frequency is increasing and, if so, why? Chronic fatigue syndrome is clearly related to several vaguely defined syndromes, both epidemic and sporadic, described in the medical literature since the late nineteenth century. The concept of a postviral fatigue syndrome is likely to be a valid clinical entity as old as viruses and man. Postviral neuromyasthenia, as it was called by some in the older medical literature, seemingly was either common or prolonged but not both. Postviral fatigue in its common form was self-limited and only rarely was it prolonged. If epidemic, then it was geographically confined to a small locality and never generalized to an entire nation. CFS, as defined in the opening paragraph, now appears to be common, prolonged, epidemic, and generalized across national boundaries, which suggests an immediate difference with past descriptions.

An apparent rise in cases, probably from the 1970s, both in this country and overseas, suggests a pandemic. Random national surveys by this author of groups of patients who joined CEBV support groups in 1986 show an exponential case production curve beginning in the early to mid-1970s with 70 percent of patients becoming ill in the last five years. The fidelity of this survey data from region to region, as well as the rate of rise established well before media interest began in 1985, argues in favor of its validity. If valid then there may be more than one interpretation, including the possibility that CFS is about five years in length for most patients, which would produce a similar curve to the one observed. At the moment no one can know the truth with certainty. One possibility may be that a new agent has been creating a pandemic of CFS since the early 1970s, superimposed on a constant baseline production of similar-appearing cases of postviral fatigue syndrome. Postviral fatigue, or neuromyasthenia, then, represents a much older, and probably generic, problem. What is more far-fetched than this view is that we could have, in the closing years of the twentieth century, such a poor clinical concept of an "old" disease that is as common and impressive as CFS is today. How could we have missed this often impressive disorder for so long? Today's CFS patients can easily write books on a disorder that has generated only a handful of research papers in a hundred years. Too many good clinicians have stated, "I've never seen anything quite like this," and perhaps they are right.

Another important question concerns how to make the diagnosis of CFS/CFIDS. When considering a diagnosis of CFS, one is often faced with a group of alternate diagnoses, the so-called differential diagnoses. A recent publication has given a rather extensive list of other diagnoses that, while possible in a given case, have not proven to be very commonly found in the experience of most referral clinicians who deal with CFS. That so few patients have been found to have "other, more plausible explanations" for their symptoms is remarkable and attests to the validity of CFS as a clinical entity. There are, however, several related disorders that are most often considered and that may not, for a variety of reasons, be easily dismissed. In order of frequency they are:

1. Depression or related mood disorders
2. Somatization disorder
3. Fibromyalgia
4. Constitutional deficit since childhood/adolescence
5. Allergies and other sensitivities
6. Multiple sclerosis
7. Neuromuscular disorders of uncertain cause
8. Acute infectious mono with prolonged recovery
9. Autoimmune disorders

The relationship of CFS to the above disorders may be closer than the usual list of differential diagnoses. Many patients given a diagnosis from the above list are just CFS patients by another name, or vice versa. It is likely that similar pathophysiologic mechanisms are at work to explain some of the symptom similarities. There may also be genetic and other factors that predispose people to disorders that possess related pathophysiologies. Finally, it is possible that CFS itself can produce in some patients a clinical picture identical to some of the above diagnoses. Despite the admittedly complex relationship of CFS to the above disorders, the usual case of CFS can be differentiated on clinical and other grounds and may have unique and, more recently, even novel causes.

Serious obstacles to further progress are lack of a consensus over case definition and political divisions in our medical research centers over whether this problem even exists. Lack of a good case definition will quickly lead to studies of "fatigue" patients with too heterogeneous a mix of pathophysiologies to give meaningful results. A lack of coherent and reproducible studies will only fuel professional divisions. Another problem is the relative lack of rigorous and systematic clinical database collections on a large group of these patients in one place who can be followed over time. Longitudinal clinical studies will help determine separate subpopulations of these patients. Analysis of subpopulations will be very important if patients who meet a given case definition are ill from different agents or pathophysiologic mechanisms. It is possible, however, that a case definition exists in which the great majority of patients are ill from a single agent or basic mechanism. As discussed above, it is almost certain that several pathophysiologic mechanisms exist in CFS that also operate in many other diseases. Insights gained from the study of CFS will likely have "spin-offs" for a number of other both organic and apparently psychiatric disorders often equated or associated with CFS.

# Appendix C

# Summary of Current CFS Research From the National Institutes of Health

*Overview of the Chronic Fatigue Syndrome Research Program*
*National Institute of Allergy and Infectious Diseases*
*National Institutes of Health*

**NIAID**    **National Institute of Allergy and Infectious Diseases**

## WHAT IS NIAID DOING ABOUT CFS?

- Since 1986, the National Institute of Allergy and Infectious Diseases (NIAID), a component of the National Institutes of Health (NIH), has provided grants to researchers around the country to investigate many aspects of CFS and CFS-like illnesses. Approximately 80 percent of NIAID's budget supports research conducted by scientists at universities, medical schools, and private research institutions, primarily within the United States. NIAID estimates it will spend $4.8 million on CFS research in fiscal year 1996.

- NIAID continues to support multidisciplinary research projects on the illness through its CFS Cooperative Research Centers program (see "University-Based CFS Research Supported by NIAID"), established in 1991.
- NIAID's on-campus CFS research team has begun a new placebo-controlled CFS treatment trial in collaboration with physicians at The Johns Hopkins University School of Medicine. The study is based on recent findings by the Hopkins group suggesting a link between CFS and neurally mediated hypotension. (See "The CFS Research Program in Bethesda.")
- In the fall of 1996, NIAID, together with several other NIH institutes, released the sixth in a series of announcements inviting scientists to submit grant applications proposing novel approaches to study the pathophysiology of the disease. Investigators will be encouraged to address research gaps, such as CFS in pregnancy and adolescents, and emerging areas of study, such as neurally mediated hypotension.
- NIAID's revision of its publication on CFS for health professionals is nearing completion. Its availability will be announced on the NIAID home page on the World Wide Web.

## WHAT IS CFS?

Chronic fatigue syndrome (CFS) is characterized by six months or more of profound persistent or relapsing fatigue that is unrelieved by rest. This fatigue occurs together with other symptoms, most often recurrent sore throats, muscle pain, multijoint pain, tender lymph nodes, new types or patterns of headaches, and neuropsychological complaints such as impaired memory or concentration.

Many distinguished scientists throughout the United States

and elsewhere are studying CFS. So far, there is no published evidence indicating that CFS is contagious or transmissible through casual or intimate contact. Unlike contagious-disease cases, the vast majority of CFS cases appear sporadically rather than in clusters. In addition, large population-based surveys conducted by the Centers for Disease Control and Prevention have found no increased risk for CFS among members of households in which a person with CFS resides.

The cause of CFS is unknown. To date, extensive research efforts by many different scientists have failed to find evidence that a retrovirus or any other single virus or other infectious agent causes CFS, or that a unique set of immune system alterations is specific to this condition. Research now points toward multiple factors rather than a single factor as causing the neuroendocrine or other global physiological disturbances seen in CFS.

## UNIVERSITY-BASED CFS RESEARCH SUPPORTED BY NIAID

All research grant applications received by NIAID are reviewed by two independent panels of nongovernment scientists. The first review is by an initial review group convened by NIH or NIAID. NIH established an initial review group called a Special Emphasis Panel for CFS to ensure that CFS grant applications receive appropriate scientific consideration by nongovernment experts knowledgeable about CFS. The second review is by the institute's National Advisory Allergy and Infectious Diseases Council, a group of scientists and laypersons that meets regularly to advise the institute on research funding, priorities, and policies. Only those applications deemed highly meritorious are funded. Within NIAID, the Division of Microbiology and Infectious Diseases oversees the administration of CFS research projects.

Current funded studies focus on prevalence, diagnosis, laboratory and clinical markers (including viruses and cytokines), natural history, cognitive impairment, physiologic function, and physiological response to exertion.

In 1991, NIAID established the CFS Cooperative Research Centers (CFS-CRCs) program to encourage multidisciplinary research to understand the cause(s) and physiological bases of CFS, including studies of virologic and immunologic factors for their roles in the illness. In 1995, the recompetition for the CFS-CRCs resulted in the award of two center grants to the University of Washington in Seattle (206-521-1935) and the University of Medicine and Dentistry in Newark, New Jersey (201-982-2552). The centers continue to focus their research on the pathogenesis of the disease and include novel approaches, such as comparing twins, one with CFS and one without, to elucidate risk factors for the illness. Ongoing studies also seek to determine the relationship between exercise, physiological changes, and symptoms in CFS patients.

The centers also conduct pilot projects to facilitate rapid testing of new hypotheses and approaches. To date, NIAID has supported twenty-four pilot projects, two of which formed the basis for successful independent research grants. Regular meetings of CFS-CRC investigators encourage collaboration and promote research progress.

NIAID has undertaken five initiatives to foster CFS research and has organized five workshops on research issues in CFS. The goal of these workshops has been to promote sound research approaches and to foster fruitful collaborations among scientists.

## THE CFS RESEARCH PROGRAM IN BETHESDA

NIAID scientists working at the NIH campus in Bethesda, Maryland, began research on a CFS-like illness in 1979. (The syndrome was not named CFS until 1988.) Stephen Straus, M.D., a virologist and chief of NIAID's Laboratory of Clinical Investigation (LCI), coauthored one of the first papers to delineate the clinical, virologic, and immunologic features of the syndrome. Later, the LCI group published results of the first controlled therapeutic trial for CFS. Although this study demonstrated that acyclovir, a drug selected because of its ability to inhibit the activity of Epstein-Barr virus (EBV), was *not* an effective treatment for CFS, the study represented the first prospective analysis of CFS patients and established the standard for CFS treatment trials. Based on more recent studies by Dr. Straus's group and their collaborators showing that CFS patients have lower-than-normal levels of circulating and urinary cortisol—the so-called stress hormone—the LCI group has undertaken and nearly completed a placebo-controlled therapeutic trial of low doses of oral hydrocortisone.

The LCI researchers have collaborated with many experts in other scientific disciplines both inside and outside NIH to explore diverse avenues of CFS research. CFS patients have been compared with patients who have other chronic illnesses and with healthy people in order to better understand the epidemiology, natural history, clinical features, and pathogenesis of CFS.

Other collaborative investigations involving the LCI group have included the following:

- *Viruses:* Studies of EBV serology and virology, herpesviruses (including HHV 6), retroviruses, and enteroviruses. These studies are part of a large body of data that to date have found no evidence of a single viral agent as the cause of CFS.
- *Immunology:* Studies of cytokine levels, cytokine release from cells, interferon 2'5'-oligoadenylate synthetase, immune complexes, and lymphocyte phenotyping.
- *Physiology:* Studies of muscles and muscle fatigue, cognitive function, neuroendocrine levels, rehabilitation, and the current trial of hydrocortisone therapy.

- *Epidemiology:* Studies comparing CFS cases derived by different case definitions. Investigations looking for overlap with other illnesses have found no relationship to Sjögren's syndrome or postpolio syndrome but there is a recognized overlap with fibromyalgia.

Scientists at the Johns Hopkins University School of Medicine recently reported a possible link between CFS and a blood-pressure-regulation disorder called neurally mediated hypotension, which sometimes responds to drug therapy. LCI researchers and the Hopkins scientists are collaborating on a large placebo-controlled, double-blind treatment study using fludrocortisone (Florinef) in an attempt to confirm the preliminary findings. Patients can call 1-800-772-5464 (in the Washington, D.C., area, 301-496-9054, extension 659) for further details; physicians can call 301-496-9054, extension 658.

The CFS projects carried out by Dr. Straus and his colleagues receive funding from the budget of NIAID's Division of Intramural Research. The scientific progress of NIAID's intramural program is regularly reviewed by an outside Board of Scientific Counselors.

## ADVISORY COUNCIL REVIEW OF NIAID'S CFS PROGRAM

In September 1995, a subcommittee of the NIAID Advisory Council met to discuss the CFS program supported by NIAID. For this review, the membership of the subcommittee was supplemented by scientists knowledgeable in the areas of infectious diseases and CFS. Seven scientists whose research reflects current concepts and aspects of CFS pathophysiology were also invited to present reviews of their research and to answer questions from the review panel.

The intramural program was praised for the depth and

extent of its research and for the involvement of investigators both at other NIH institutes and extramurally.

The subcommittee concluded that the extramural program's multidisciplinary approach and interactions with other NIH institutes and Public Health Service agencies are important and should continue. It recognized the depth and extent of the research conducted by NIAID-supported scientists and their collaborators. Among the subcommittee's recommendations was the suggestion that investigators continue to think of CFS as a symptom complex and not a single disease, thus allowing them to consider multiple causative factors.

NIAID, a component of the National Institutes of Health, supports research on AIDS, tuberculosis, and other infectious diseases, as well as allergies and immunology. NIH is an agency of the U.S. Public Health Service, U.S. Department of Health and Human Services.

# APPENDIX D

# Where to Go for Help

## PATIENT NETWORKS

The following CFS organizations are the largest in the country. They publish newsletters and can help you find a support group in your area.

National Chronic Fatigue Syndrome and Fibromyalgia Association (NCFSFA)
P.O. Box 18426
Kansas City, MO 64133
(816) 313-2000
(For information from the NCFSFA, see page 225.)

The CFIDS Association of America, Inc.
P.O. Box 220398
Charlotte, NC 28222-0398
(800) 442-3437
(For information from the CFIDS Association of America, see page 229.)

## GOVERNMENT AGENCIES THAT PROVIDE INFORMATION

These agencies send free CFS information packets:

National Institute of Allergy and Infectious Diseases
Office of Communications,
9000 Rockville Pike
Building 31, Room 7A50
Bethesda, MD 20892
(301) 496-5717

Centers for Disease Control and Prevention
Mail Stop G-18
Atlanta, GA 30333
(404) 639-1338

# INFORMATION FROM THE NATIONAL CHRONIC FATIGUE SYNDROME AND FIBROMYALGIA ASSOCIATION

The founders of the National Chronic Fatigue Syndrome Association, an all-volunteer, 501(c)(3) nonprofit organization, incorporated in February 1988, first began their educational efforts in 1985. In 1988, the NCFSA was formed to educate and inform the public about the nature and impact of chronic fatigue syndrome and related disorders. In 1993, the board of directors voted unanimously to add fibromyalgia to its educational efforts. Thus, the name of the organization was changed to the National Chronic Fatigue Syndrome and Fibromyalgia Association.

From our beginning, we sought cautious and competent help from the scientific community. The primary focus of the organization is to offer scientifically accurate information for chronic fatigue syndrome and fibromyalgia. Such efforts are accomplished by relying on information published by the National Institutes of Health, Centers for Disease Control and Prevention, various peer-reviewed, scientifically accurate, medical publications, and from reliable medical advisers. Accomplishments include:

1995

- Cosponsor, with the Regional Arthritis Center and St. Luke's Hospital, a one-day seminar titled "Fibromyalgia: Understanding a Diverse Disease" with over 560 people attending
- Association president Orvalene Prewitt assisted in planning and participating in a half-day session on chronic fatigue syndrome held on the National Institutes of Health campus, Bethesda, Maryland, focusing on the current knowledge and research findings in CFS.

**1994**

- Appointment of association president Orvalene Prewitt by secretary of health, Dr. Donna Shalala, to serve on the National Advisory Allergy and Infectious Disease Council of the National Institutes of Health, and to be one of four lay consultants to the Health and Human Service Chronic Fatigue Syndrome Interagency Coordinating Committee (CFSICC), comprised of representatives from the NIH, CDC, SSA, and FDA
- Sponsored workshops on "Dealing with the Diverse Symptoms of Chronic Fatigue Syndrome and Fibromyalgia"

**1993**

- The association was featured in Harvard Medical School's September 1993 issue of *Harvard Health Letter.*

**1992**

- The association's annually sponsored "Chronic Fatigue Syndrome Awareness Month" concluded at the White House for a meeting with First Lady Barbara Bush.

**1991**

- Cofounder and President Orvalene Prewitt was recognized by President and Mrs. Bush for her volunteer efforts in the "Thousand Points of Light" program.

**1990**

- The association's reputation for providing accurate information resulted in the organization being recognized in the October 1990 issue of *Consumer Reports.*

## SERVICES OFFERED BY NCFSFA

### Patient Education

- twenty-four-hour information line
- assist our two chapters, National Chronic Fatigue

Syndrome and Fibromyalgia Association in Topeka, Kansas, and the National Chronic Fatigue Syndrome and Fibromyalgia Association in Wichita, Kansas

- monthly support group meetings
- newsletter (usually quarterly) that offers scientifically accurate information
- sponsor Chronic Fatigue Syndrome Awareness Month each year in March
- provide referrals to support groups, phone contacts, physicians (We work with over 400 support groups and phone contacts in the United States and abroad.)
- educate patients to become partners in their health care and stress the importance to patients of obtaining accurate information
- advise members of research studies available for patient participation
- provide educational materials including audio- and videotapes, eleven brochures on various aspects of the illness, patient and physician packets, information packets on how to start a reputable support group, etc.
- maintain advocacy program with state and federal officials

## Medical Professionals

- attempt to build stronger communication between physicians and patients
- attempt to keep medical community informed of new publications, especially those from the National Institutes of Health, Centers for Disease Control and Prevention, and Public Health Service
- respond to inquiries for information and act as a referral service for physicians nationwide and abroad
- hold educational forums, which often offer CME credits and encourage grand rounds
- utilize medical professionals as advisers to our association
- help fund educational forums

Research
- maintain an advocacy program to encourage continued government funding for research
- rely on peer-review research to enable us to offer reliable educational materials to inquirers
- partially funded five research surveys on various aspects of chronic fatigue syndrome
- award specified research funds of which distributions are subject to a grant application process and peer review by a medical advisory committee

# INFORMATION FROM THE CFIDS ASSOCIATION OF AMERICA

The suffering inflicted by CFS can be alleviated only through education, enlightened public policy, and research—the three areas in which the CFIDS Association of America leads the nation. These association-sponsored programs have brought early and impressive progress and are essential to the battle against CFIDS.

The CFIDS Association of America is the nation's leading charitable organization dedicated to conquering chronic fatigue and immune dysfunction syndrome (CFIDS). Since 1987 its efforts to expand education and research have greatly enhanced understanding of this complex and debilitating illness.

Each year the association responds to tens of thousands of requests for free information and conducts hundreds of mass mailings to persons with CFIDS (PWCs), family members and friends of PWCs, medical professionals, government officials, and the media. In addition to its quarterly publication, *The CFIDS Chronicle,* the association publishes and distributes various informational literature about CFIDS, including newsletters for support group leaders and young PWCs. The association maintains the most complete collection available of books, medical and media articles, and video- and audiotapes about CFIDS. Topics, title listings, and prices are available by calling the Resource Line at (704) 365-2343 or by visiting the association on-line at http://cfids.org/cfids.

Through its public policy program, the association has engaged the federal government in the study of CFIDS. Between 1990 and 1995, federal dollars spent on CFIDS research more than tripled, and government-funded research investigations have yielded valuable information about the illness. These advances are due largely to the commitment of the association and its members, who want to elicit a focused scientific response to CFIDS from the federal government.

The international multidisciplinary research effort to identify the cause(s) of and effective treatments for CFIDS has been stimulated by the association's $2 million investment in its peer-reviewed medical research program. Several projects funded by the association have gone on to compete successfully for federal grants, while others have yielded important pilot study data for further investigation.

---

GREGG CHARLES FISHER is the author of the original groundbreaking edition of *Chronic Fatigue Syndrome: A Victim's Guide to Understanding, Treating & Coping with This Debilitating Illness*. A fifteen-year survivor of CFS, he is nationally recognized in the CFS community and has appeared on numerous radio and television programs, including *Connie Martinson Talks Books* out of Los Angeles, *CNBC* with Dr. Georgia Whitkin, and *Mother's Day* with Joan Lunden. He lives on Long Island, New York.

# Index